Praise for
TOXIN-FREE
BODY & HOME
Starting Today

"Dr. Lee Cowden and Connie Strasheim have written an extremely important book. The toxins in our environment are increasing daily, and people must protect themselves from heavy metals, insecticides, pesticides, plastics, phthalates, GMO-type foods, and electromagnetic fields that come from things like Wi-Fi and cordless phones—just to mention a few. The total toxic burden that most people have in their bodies is not only causing them enormous symptoms—from insomnia to headaches and cardiac problems—but is also impacting their vital DNA. This book educates you while at the same time giving you simple, easy solutions to implement. It can literally save your life!"

—STEPHEN T. SINATRA, MD, FACC
Founder of HeartMDinstitute.com, and co-author of
The Great Cholesterol Myth and *Earthing:*
The Most Important Health Discovery Ever?

"This isn't just a book on detoxification; it's a guide to finally getting well. Cowden and Strasheim do an excellent job enlightening you to the hidden toxins in your home, environment and body. Until you get rid of those, you'll never get well. Buy this book!"

—SUZY COHEN, RPH, bestselling author of
The 24-Hour Pharmacist, Diabetes Without Drugs and
Drug Muggers: Which Medications are Robbing Your Body of Essential
Nutrients and How to Restore Them (DearPharmacist.com)

"Thirty years ago, I started writing books about how to reverse disease by finding and correcting its underlying causes. Today, we find ourselves in an even more toxic, disease-ridden world, more desperately in need of truth about the causes of disease, as well as solutions for it. This book, *Create a Toxin-Free Body & Home Starting Today* by Dr. Lee Cowden and Connie Strasheim, will introduce the reader to toxicity-related causes of illness in the home and outdoor environment. The solutions are presented in a format that is easy to understand and implement. *Create a Toxin-Free Body & Home Starting Today* will help readers to understand that they alone have the power to reverse and prevent toxicity-related illness, and gain the necessary knowledge that will enable them to become too smart to fail in their quest for wellness."

—SHERRY ROGERS, MD, bestselling author of
How to Cure Diabetes and *Detoxify or Die*
(PrestigePublishing.com)

ACIM

The Journey to Wellness Book Series

Create a
Toxin-Free
Body & Home
Starting Today

W. Lee Cowden, MD, MD(H)
Connie Strasheim

ACIM Press

Books may be purchased in bulk by contacting the publisher and author at:
ACIMConnect.com

Cover Design: Nick Zelinger, NZ Graphics
Interior Design: Rebecca Finkel, F + P Graphic Design
Publisher: ACIM Press
Editor: John Maling, Editing By John
Publishing Consultant: Judith Briles, The Book Shepherd

First edition
Library of Congress Catalog Number: 2014939260
ISBN paperback: 978-0-9961004-0-3
eISBN: 978-0-9961004-1-0
CIP on file

1. Health   2. Environmental Living   3. Holisitc Health

Printed in the USA

Contents

Foreword

As the inventor of chelation—or detoxification—therapy, I am sometimes referred to in the medical community as the Father of Chelation. Besides having treated many thousands of patients for health conditions related to environmental toxicity, I have owned my own mineral lab, tested hundreds of thousands of people for heavy metal toxins, and developed nutritional supplements.

My experience as a holistic doctor who specializes in chelation therapy, along with my experience as a mineral lab owner, consultant and supplement developer, has led me to believe that environmental toxins are the foremost cause of most chronic and degenerative diseases today. This belief has been substantiated by my own recovery from a lifetime of severe chronic illness caused by environmental toxins.

It is essential that we remove toxins from our bodies and homes in order to live long, healthy lives. And I am thrilled to endorse this wonderful collaborative effort between Dr. Lee

Cowden and Connie Strasheim because they have put forth a practical "do-it-yourself" book of detoxification strategies that will help you maintain health and avoid a multitude of chronic degenerative diseases caused by environmental toxicity. I believe this book will help thousands, if not millions of people.

I initially became interested in detoxification when I realized that toxicity was the main cause of my own health problems, which I had struggled with from my birth until fifteen years ago.

As a child and during my formative years, I often had high fevers with no known cause. I suffered from serious heart problems, including heart block, which caused skipped heartbeats and arrhythmias, so I couldn't participate in sports or even swim one pool lap. My body didn't make sufficient stomach acid so I couldn't absorb much-needed minerals like magnesium, and I was sensitive to most foods. I suffered from severe neck spasms and back pain. My testicles were also much smaller than normal and did not produce sperm. One of my kidneys was injured and doctors wanted to remove it, but I refused and so wound up with chronic kidney disease. In medical school, I couldn't climb a flight of steps without having heart failure. I was a total basket case.

Part of my suffering was due to the heavy metal toxins that I had been exposed to because of incompetent dentists who had filled my mouth many times with toxic mercury fillings. After receiving one particular round of fillings, I spent the better part of the next year in bed. I was told I had narcolepsy, but it was really the effects of amalgam poisoning that had made me very sick.

So I have experienced firsthand the effects of environmental toxins and suffered a lifetime of illness because of what I did not know back then about toxins. However, unlike today, at the time that I was sick there were no good environmentally savvy doctors around to treat me, so I had to discover, through trial and error, what was causing my symptoms and how to resolve them.

Now at age 78, I'm the healthiest that I've ever been in my life, and it's because of what I've learned about detoxification.

Chelation, or intravenous heavy metal removal, opened the first door to wellness for me, followed by ultraviolet blood irradiation and ozone therapy—all of which cleanse the blood and body of harmful toxins. To this day, I take toxin binders and do detoxification therapies. I've been taking oral EDTA daily (a heavy metal binder) over the past 25 years and I feel better and better all the time.

These days, I provide consulting services on detoxification and other health issues to thousands of patients and doctors worldwide, through the Gordon Research Institute: *GordonResearch.com.* I am also the creator of the FIGHT program, which stands for "Food, Infection, Genetics, Hormones, and Toxins." All of these factor into wellness, and must be addressed for full health to occur.

I recommend, as part of the FIGHT program, key detoxification supplements such as Bio En'R-G'y C and ZeoGold Enhanced, which I have designed and developed to eliminate a variety of pollutants from the body.

I spent in excess of $80,000 to research the vitamin C product, Bio En'R-G'y C, and successfully proved that this product increases cellular energy and enables nutrients to get into the cells. The cells cannot eliminate toxins or uptake nutrients without energy, so I wanted to create a vitamin C product that would do this. These are just two supplements that aid in detoxification. More are described in this book, as well as on my website.

I got my life back by detoxifying my body, and it's because of my personal experience and experience with many others that I highly recommend this book. It offers a crucial message of hope to those who are afflicted with a variety of health problems, as well as to those who simply want to prevent illness.

If my experience doesn't convince you about the impact that environmental toxins have upon the body, consider this: A 2007-2008 research study by the Environmental Working Group (EWR) (www.ewr.org) proved that all babies are born with as many as 232 neurotoxic chemical compounds inside their bodies, before they have even been exposed to life outside the womb. If there are that many toxic chemicals inside a newborn, imagine how many pollutants have accumulated in an adult who has been on this planet for 30, 40 or 60 years!

Other studies have confirmed the EWR study. For instance, one study, conducted at the California Institute of Technology, revealed that newborns have anywhere from 1,000 to 2,000 times more lead in their bones than babies that were born before the industrial age. And another study, conducted at Harvard, revealed that bone lead levels correlate with the amount of lead in other parts of the body, such as the kidneys, eyes and liver. This means that it's not just the bones that have high amounts of lead, but other parts of the body, too.

And then nurses vaccinate these babies, even when the instructions on vaccine package inserts advise against vaccination if the child is sick. But how can babies not be sick when they have 1,000 to 2,000 times the amount of lead in their bodies as their ancestors?

Then there are the holistic integrative medical doctors who can verify, through their experiences with thousands of patients, how toxins are poisoning us, and causing the majority of chronic, degenerative diseases of today, such as Alzheimer's, Parkinson's, multiple sclerosis, fibromyalgia, chronic fatigue syndrome, and so on.

For instance, one prominent physician, Dr. Philip Landrigan, a pediatrician and Dean of Health at the Mt. Sinai School of Medicine in New York, used to test his patients for toxins. He reports that he has never seen a single child who hasn't tested positive for harmful environmental contaminants such as bisphenol-A, dioxins, mercury and other chemical pollutants. When environmentally trained doctors lower the levels of contaminants in their patients, the patients often recover, even if they have failed all prior treatments.

When I owned Mineral Lab in Hayward, California, I saw hundreds of thousands of test results proving that people everywhere in the United States are full of lead and mercury.

If more people realized this—and, for example, that newborns are a chemical time bomb and that we all have toxins that are harming our health and causing degenerative diseases such as Alzheimer's, autoimmune and heart disease—they might take steps to remove them. If they knew how greatly these toxins were harming their health, they might spend some of their hard-earned money on treatment strategies to remove the toxins, instead of saving for a new car.

If you still aren't convinced about the dangers of toxins, consider Dr. William Rea, a vascular surgeon, who took over part of a Marriott hotel and converted it into a haven for chemically-sensitive people. He discovered that whenever people with any kind of health condition would stay there, they became virtually symptom-free. This in itself proves that we environmental doctors aren't crazy when we tell you that detoxification matters!

Unfortunately, we can't stop the polluters of this planet, but I have high hopes that through books like *Create a Toxin-Free Body & Home Starting Today*, and by coming up with ways to make man tougher, with quality nutritional supplements and detoxification strategies, we can become more resilient to these toxins. Thank heavens, Dr. Cowden's and Connie's approach to detoxification is truly a practical one, and details about how to easily and effectively remove environmental contaminants from your body and home have all been carefully laid out in this book.

Their strategies are also innovative. For instance, Dr. Cowden has simplified homeopathy and added laser to his detoxification protocols and in so doing has saved many lives. He has also put unique ideas together about detoxification and healing that no other physician has.

We can't run away from toxic exposures but we can reduce their effects upon us by implementing the strategies in this book. Physicians like Dr. Cowden and I simply have to convince you that you aren't wasting your money when you purchase things like vitamin C, oral chelation, zeolite or other detoxification remedies. You may not feel an immediate effect from them, but by taking them, your body will have a greater ability to handle all of the toxins to which it's exposed daily, and over time, you will be healthier and happier.

We all live with limited information, and even those of us who believe ourselves to be healthy may be candidates for future illness because of the damage that toxins can do to the body. Thankfully, it is possible to reverse such damage. I spent my life overcoming significant health challenges, and in so doing, I have paved a way for others to become well.

In a toxic world, we need toxin-removal strategies in order to live life to the fullest. This book delivers those strategies and gives me hope that, even while the environment is frightening, we can yet remain healthy and strong and thrive, becoming the "invincible" humans that we need to be.

—GARRY GORDON, MD, DO, MD(H)

Garry Gordon, MD, DO, MD(H), author of *The Chelation Answer* and *The Definitive Guide to Longevity Medicine*, advisor to The American Board of Chelation Therapy

Preface

In today's toxic, hurried and stressful world, most people's goal is simply to survive. In such a world, where weariness, worry and pain are the norm, wellness has come to mean, for most, an absence of symptoms or mere functionality.

But what if, in our journey towards wellness, we are not meant to just survive, but rather, to thrive? What if we could have life abundant, in body, mind and spirit, simply by applying certain key principles to our lives? Imagine having a strong, balanced and energetic body; a sound, peaceful mind; a joyful, positive and loving spirit; and a prosperous, restful and productive life.

This book is the first in a series that's designed to provide you with the tools that you need to be whole and to embrace life more fully.

We, the authors of this book, believe that these are the fruits of the wellness journey and can be attained by most people if they are just given the proper tools.

Abundance and health aren't just meant for those who were lucky enough to have emotionally balanced and loving parents, perfect genes, material wealth or the right connections. Though life may present incredible challenges to our well-being, with the right tools we can not only overcome those challenges but prosper and be in excellent health.

The tools that lead us down the road to optimum wellness can be divided into different categories, according to their function and role in bringing us to a place of wholeness. Indeed, when we are made whole at every level of our being, we become fully equipped to fulfill our destinies, no matter the circumstances that befall us. This book presents the first of the tools necessary for health and an abundant life.

We live in a world where environmental toxins are increasingly contaminating our bodies, homes and workplaces. At best these toxins slow us down and prevent us from functioning optimally, and at worst they disable us with chronic illness.

The good news is we can identify and remove the influence of many of these toxins upon our bodies, homes and other places where we spend the most time.

When these places become clean, and our bodies are then detoxified, the other tools of wellness, which will be described in other books in *The Journey to Wellness* series, can work more effectively to bring about wholeness—in body, mind and spirit.

If you already struggle with health problems or are very sick, following most, if not all, of the strategies recommended in this book may be important for your recovery. If you are mostly well or just dealing with a minor health problem or two, you may be able to get away with doing only some of them.

In any case, and no matter where you fall along the spectrum of wellness, we recommend implementing as many of the strategies found in this book as you can—without putting undue stress on yourself if you can't do them all or apply them perfectly. Sometimes the stress of feeling like you have to do everything right can become a greater stress upon your body than the stress that toxins cause, so it's important to consider carefully those strategies that will be most helpful to you for your particular situation.

We believe that as your body and home become unburdened by the weight of these toxins, you will feel progressively happier, healthier and more alive—perhaps more so than ever before!

This book is the first in a series that's designed to provide you with the tools that you need to be whole and to embrace life more fully. It is written from two perspectives: first, from that of an internationally renowned integrative medical doctor who has treated thousands of patients with a myriad of health conditions, and who has extensive knowledge and wisdom about holistic wellness; and secondly, from a medical writer who has experienced severe chronic illness firsthand and learned, through a decade of being "in the trenches," what it takes to prosper and be well in body, mind and spirit.

May the information enlighten, inspire and divinely guide you in your wellness journey!

— **William Lee Cowden, MD**
and **Connie Strasheim**

Introduction

Toxins and Their Harmful Impact upon Us

Many of us don't realize the detrimental impact of environmental toxins upon our lives until we begin to remove them from our bodies and homes.

Only then do we discover that toxins are the reason we have been profoundly fatigued or wandering around in a fog, forgetting appointments; or enduring recurring headaches, backaches and stomachaches.

We live in a world where environmental toxins are increasingly contaminating our bodies, homes and workplaces. At best, these toxins slow us down and prevent us from functioning optimally, and at worst they disable us with chronic illness.

Only then do we learn that toxins are the reason we are contentious with our friends and family; suffering from hormonal imbalances; or tossing and turning at night in a fitful slumber.

Only then do we see that our woes aren't just the result of the normal aches and pains of daily living, and that popping some anti-inflammatory drug or sleeping pill or chugging down big mugs of coffee are coping mechanisms that never get to the root of the problem.

But as we eliminate toxins, our minds begin to operate with clarity and sharpness; the creaks and kinks in our joints and muscles begin to disappear, and suddenly we realize that toxins were a major part of what was keeping us from total health.

For some of us, detoxifying our body and environment simply brings about a new awareness of wellness; of awakening in the morning with pep and vitality; of a new ability to accomplish tasks, or a zest for life that previously did not exist. And yet, for others of us, toxin removal is the difference between being bedridden and being able to make it to a job.

All of us are affected by toxins. Nobody in modern-day society is exempt from their influence because they abound in the air, water and food supply, as well as in our homes, household products, cars, and industrial substances and materials that we come into contact with daily. Such toxins include heavy metals, biotoxins (which are produced by harmful microbes), industrial contaminants, radiation, chemicals and pharmaceutical drugs, as well as many others, and they harm the body in a multitude of ways.

Toxins disrupt enzyme and hormonal systems; alter metabolic processes, brain chemistry and digestion. They contaminate cells and cause them to retain waste at the same time that they prevent them from using nutrients and oxygen. They keep the brain and body from effectively making and using energy, and they harm and cause disease in the body's organs so that they cease to function properly. They then cause symptoms and illnesses that can affect every aspect of our minds, bodies and spirits. If our minds are impaired by toxicity, it also becomes very difficult for us to function at an optimal level spiritually. In this book, we will describe in greater detail how toxins negatively impact the body and what can be done to remove their influence so that we can function in the manner in which we were designed.

All of us are affected by toxins. Nobody in modern-day society is exempt from their influence because they abound in the air, water and food supply, as well as in our homes, household products, cars, and industrial substances and materials that we come into contact with daily.

For the purposes of this book, we will be mostly focusing upon the influence that toxins have upon the body, but it's important to note that the body operates in unison with the mind and spirit, and when one is affected, the other two often are also. So toxins create dysfunction and chaos at every level. As long as they plague us, we will struggle to survive, never mind thrive. Therefore, toxin removal is the first essential tool for creating optimal wellness so that we can thrive amidst the barrage of air, water and food toxins to which we are exposed daily.

The Bathtub Analogy

Suppose the bathtub in the image below represents your body, and the faucets represent all of the factors, positive and negative, that can get poured into it and which will determine its overall state of wellness.

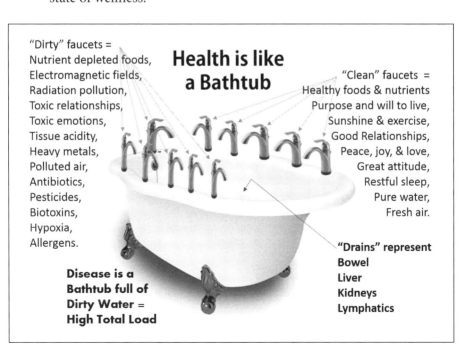

"Dirty" faucets =
Nutrient depleted foods,
Electromagnetic fields,
Radiation pollution,
Toxic relationships,
Toxic emotions,
Tissue acidity,
Heavy metals,
Polluted air,
Antibiotics,
Pesticides,
Biotoxins,
Hypoxia,
Allergens.

Health is like a Bathtub

"Clean" faucets =
Healthy foods & nutrients
Purpose and will to live,
Sunshine & exercise,
Good Relationships,
Peace, joy, & love,
Great attitude,
Restful sleep,
Pure water,
Fresh air.

"Drains" represent
Bowel
Liver
Kidneys
Lymphatics

Disease is a
Bathtub full of
Dirty Water =
High Total Load

If the bathtub were to represent a chronically ill person, it would be overloaded with toxins to the point that it could no longer manage to eliminate those toxins, and there would be dirty water overflowing and spilling onto the floor. The dirty water would represent physical symptoms, so a bathtub of dirty water represents disease. Notice that this word can be broken down into two parts: "dis" and "ease." When the body is sick, it is not at ease! When we can move away from "dis," we become at "ease," and when we are at ease, we are at peace and feel good.

The factors that cause too much dirty water to flow into the bathtub and spill over include: nutrient-depleted foods, electromagnetic pollution, antibiotics, heavy metals, radiation, pesticides, biotoxins, allergens, and toxic emotions, among others. Some of these factors, such as toxic relationships and emotions, will be described in later books in this series, since this book focuses only on environmental toxins in the body and home.

The factors that cause too much dirty water to flow into the bathtub and spill over include: nutrient-depleted foods, electromagnetic pollution, antibiotics, heavy metals, radiation, pesticides, biotoxins, allergens, antibiotics and toxic emotions.

Note the clean-water faucets on the right side of the bathtub. These represent the detoxification or healing agents that you want flowing into your tub to replace the dirty water there. The clean-water faucets represent things such as a positive attitude, healthy diet, fresh air, good relationships, peace, joy, love, restful sleep and so on. Most of those faucets are partially or even fully "turned off" in people who have health problems or symptoms of illness. So in order to heal the body, it's important to open up those faucets!

At the bottom of the bathtub are several drains. Just as it's important to fill up the bathtub with clean water and turn off as many of the dirty-water faucets as possible, it's also imperative to open up these drains so that the toxic water can flow out of the bathtub. The drains represent the bowels and other organs that remove waste from the body, including the kidneys, gallbladder, liver, urinary bladder and lymphatic system.

So the way to wellness involves first draining the bad water and turning off all the dirty-water faucets to the best of your ability, and then opening up all the good-water faucets. As you drain the bad water and pour good water into the tub, over time the water in that tub will become clearer, because now you have good water flowing in and brackish water flowing out.

If you open all of the drains enough, at some point you will see the bottom of the bathtub, because the water will be so clear! The goal of any wellness program is to have so much clean water—or healthy factors—being poured into your body that you can eventually see the bottom of the bathtub.

In this book, we will teach you how to drain harmful environmental toxins from your tub, as well as how to pour into it healthful remedies and practices to replace those that caused it to be dirty and overflowing in the first place.

Part One

Create a Toxin-Free Body

All of us have some brackish water in our bathtubs as a result of environmental toxins, whether we are sick or not. Getting these toxins out and clean water flowing in is the first essential step in the journey towards wellness. Some toxins cannot be removed from the body until they are first removed from the home, so as you are detoxifying your body we encourage you to simultaneously implement the suggestions in Part Two of this book, *Create a Toxin-Free Home*. This will ensure that your body and environment are as hospitable, clean and vibrant as can be.

TOXINS IN FOOD AND
HOW TO CHOOSE HEALTHY FOODS

Food is supposed to be the fuel that makes the body strong and healthy, but did you know that most food today is actually making people sick? This is because most of the food supply is loaded with toxins. And over time our bodies accumulate massive amounts of these toxins, as they also sift out and use the meager amounts of nutrients remaining in the food and which we need to function. No wonder many of us are puttering along at half-throttle, or suffering from a variety of chronic health conditions.

If you must shop at a conventional supermarket, it's best to shop only along the perimeter of the store, where all the fresh produce and meats are located. As the award-winning journalist Michael Pollen wrote in *Food Rules*, if your great-grandmother would not have recognized a particular food that's sold today on the shelves, you shouldn't buy it.

Just consider this: One-hundred years ago, we didn't eat antibiotics for lunch daily. We didn't ingest plastic or wax-coated fruit or chemically laden vegetables three times a day. Neither did we supplement our daily diets with hormones from animals forced to grow at four times their natural rate.

But today we do, and our food supply is being increasingly contaminated by herbicides, pesticides, antibiotics, hormones and genetically modified organisms (GMOs).

Most food that conventional grocery stores sell isn't even real food anymore. It is synthetic, chemically treated, nutrient-depleted and toxic, and many people today, even children, are developing food allergies and serious illness from eating these toxic "foods." If you have been consuming non-organic foods, their toxins toxins have been damaging your body and negatively impacting your biochemistry, even if you haven't yet developed health problems from them.

Therefore, when shopping, it's important to know how to choose healthy, non-toxic foods. This is the first important step to detoxification—ensuring that no more junk gets into your body so that you can start the process of eliminating the toxins that are already in there.

Later in this book, we describe some strategies for removing toxins that have already accumulated in the body, including those that come from food. First, though, we want to offer you some basic tips for healthful shopping and eating so that you can prevent any more harmful toxins from entering your body through your food. Again, these toxins can cause allergies and even severe illness down the road. And if you already suffer from health problems, eating clean food is probably essential for a full recovery.

It is not uncommon for young people today—children, teenagers and adults in their 20s and 30s—to develop chronic health conditions that 50 or 100 years ago were typically seen only in older people. Diabetes, mental health disorders, cancer, allergies, chronic fatigue syndrome, fibromyalgia and obesity, among other illnesses, are now rampant among both the young and old, due in part to the poor quality of our food supply.

The topic of toxic food and how to establish and maintain a diet that's healthy for your particular body type will be covered in greater depth in the second book in this series, *Foods That Fit A Unique You*. However, since toxic food is a major contributor to the body's toxic load, we briefly describe some guidelines for choosing healthy, non-toxic food here.

First, if you must shop at a conventional supermarket, it's best to shop only along the perimeter of the store, where all the fresh produce and meats are located. As the award-winning journalist Michael Pollen wrote in his book *Food Rules*, if your great-grandmother would not have recognized a particular food that's sold today on the shelves, you shouldn't buy it. This is because, unlike what our great-grandparents ate, most modern food is processed with chemical additives and preservatives and has had essential nutrients removed so that the food won't spoil on the shelf. What's left is junk food, or "fast food." But do you know why they call it fast food? Because it speeds you to your grave! So it's best to avoid eating these fake foods.

Most food that conventional grocery stores sell isn't even real food anymore. It is synthetic, chemically treated, nutrient-depleted and toxic, and many people today, even children, are developing food allergies and serious illnesses from eating these toxic "foods."

If you shop around the perimeter of the store, you'll find fresh vegetables, fruits, meats and other animal proteins, all of which are healthier than the boxed and canned foods in the middle of the store.

If you can't afford to eat organic, at least eat this non-processed, fresh food. If you are able to afford some organic food, however, we highly recommend shopping at a health food store or organic farmers' market, since most of the produce and meats found in conventional stores are genetically modified and nutrient-depleted, and have been treated with chemicals, hormones and antibiotics. These substances accumulate in the body and over time can cause hormonal imbalances, allergies, leaky gut syndrome, cancer, autoimmune illness and other diseases. Nowadays just eating your vegetables is really no longer sufficient. Those vegetables should be unadulterated if you want to experience true wellness and keep your body toxin-free.

You can often lessen your cravings for bread and other grains by cultivating a taste for other delicious foods, such as nuts and nut butters, hummus and guacamole, which you can put on veggies or apples instead of on crackers or bread.

Non-organic meats have approximately five times more pesticides than non-organic vegetables, so if you are on a strict budget and can only afford to purchase a few organic products, it's best to give priority to organic meats, and then buy organic vegetables if you have the money. This is because the pesticide content of vegetables is only about one-fifth of that found in meats, so you have to eat five times as many veggies to get the same amount of pesticide as in non-organic meat.

Non-organic meats are also laden with hormones and anti-biotics, which disrupt normal hormone function in the human body and kill off beneficial bacteria in the gut. These bacteria are the immune system's first line of defense against harmful parasites, bacteria, viruses and other organisms that enter the body through the water and food supply, so it's best to keep these healthy critters alive by not eating animal protein that has been tainted with antibiotics.

If you are able to afford some organic vegetables, it's best to spend your money first on organic root vegetables, such as carrots, beets and turnips, since non-organic root vegetables have a higher pesticide content than other types of veggies. Anything that grows in the ground has more pesticide in it than food that grows above the ground.

Sweeter fruits are more heavily sprayed with chemicals to keep the critters off them, so it's also a good idea to purchase sweet fruits organic. Conventionally harvested apples are coated with a special wax when they are picked to preserve them. This wax gets impregnated with pesticides, so if you can't afford organic apples, at the very least peel your apples before eating them.

Any fruits or vegetables that aren't organic should be washed in soap and scrubbed well to remove as many chemicals as possible.

It's Better to Go No-Grain

In the early 1900s, a dentist named Dr. Weston Price, along with Dr. Francis Pottenger, a physician who co-founded the Pottenger Sanatorium for the treatment of tuberculosis, traveled the world to find those populations that had the greatest physical and dental health. They discovered that those that never consumed grain products were the healthiest. So if you want to avoid periodontal or coronary artery disease, then don't eat grains!

Grains used to be healthy—indeed, in the Bible, bread is mentioned throughout and was a staple of some ancient societies—but modern farming, genetic manipulation and food processing methods have reduced their nutrient value and caused them to be toxic, so that many people are now allergic to them, especially wheat.

If you are used to consuming grains multiple times daily, it can be a challenge to eliminate them from your diet. Fortunately, cravings for bread and other grains can often be lessened by cultivating a taste for other delicious foods, such as nuts and nut butters, hummus and guacamole, which you can put on veggies or apples instead of on crackers or bread.

If you feel that you can't live without your grains, try some healthy gluten-free grains like brown rice, quinoa, spelt or millet, which most people tolerate better than gluten grains such as wheat. Today, health food stores sell a wide variety of gluten-free grains, pastries and cakes, made from rice, millet, spelt, almond and other types of flour. Since most corn in the United States is genetically modified, we recommend avoiding corn flour.

CLEANING UP YOUR WATER

Just as our food supply has become increasingly contaminated by toxins, so has our water supply. So if you want to detoxify your body and ensure that it remains as clean and pristine as possible, you can't be drinking dirty water.

Although it may taste okay, most U.S. city tap water today is contaminated with fluoride, chlorine, plastics, pesticides, herbicides, pharmaceutical drugs, heavy metals and other industrial contaminants, as well as parasites, viruses and other harmful micro-organisms.

Like food, the topic of healthy drinking water will be discussed more in-depth in our second book in this series, *Foods That Fit a Unique You.* Since contaminated water is a major source of toxicity, however, it's also worth mentioning here, because in order to adequately detoxify the body, it's imperative to drink and bathe only in unpolluted water.

When choosing a drinking-water filter, it's essential to use a multi-stage carbon block and/or reverse osmosis filter to remove most contaminants. Ideally, a carbon-block and KDF-resin filter should be used in the bath, too, so that you don't absorb toxins through your skin.

When choosing a drinking-water filter, it's essential to use a multi-stage carbon block and/or reverse osmosis filter to remove most contaminants. Ideally, a carbon-block and KDF-resin filter should be used in the bath, too, so that you don't absorb toxins through your skin.

If you can't afford a good water filter, which usually costs at least several hundred dollars or more, some health food stores sell reverse osmosis water, which can be stored in one-gallon or five-gallon glass containers. They also sell filters for the shower and bathtub, but unlike the multi-stage carbon block and reverse osmosis filters, some shower/bathtub filters remove only chlorine from the water. However, you can purchase carbon-block and KDF-resin shower/bathtub filters online. These will remove chlorine, most pesticides, herbicides, pharmaceuticals, solvents, plastics, heavy metals and some other industrial contaminants from the water, but not fluoride, halo-methane or all types of microbes.

It is especially important to use a filter if you live in a city, because city water is loaded with pesticides, herbicides, pharmaceutical drugs and a variety of chemical solvents. In some cities, the water is even contaminated with gasoline, which gets into the water supply when it's taken from recreational lakes that have gasoline in them because of the boaters who use the lake.

Most city water also has high amounts of chlorine and fluoride added to it. We are not aware of any study that demonstrates that adding fluoride to water is beneficial to health; however, plenty of studies show that it causes cancer, disrupts thyroid hormone production and harms the body in other ways. This is another good reason to not drink unfiltered tap water, but instead use a multi-stage, carbon-block and reverse-osmosis filter. For good-quality carbon-block and reverse-osmosis filters, visit: *MultiPure.com*.

REPLACING TOXIC PERSONAL CARE PRODUCTS WITH HEALTHY ONES

Food isn't the only thing that's toxic in your local grocery store. Nearly all personal care and makeup products contain cancer- and disease-causing chemicals that are making some of us sick.

Did you know that whatever you put onto your skin goes through your skin and into your bloodstream in the same way that the nutrients from food end up in your bloodstream? So if your personal care products aren't safe enough to eat, then you probably shouldn't be putting them on your skin either, because they end up in the same place in your body as your food.

When shopping for personal care products, it's important to read the ingredient labels to determine whether a product is toxic or not. If you don't recognize a substance in the product (if it looks like it could be a chemical, for instance), chances are it's bad for you!

Some of the most prevalent and harmful ingredients found in lotions, shampoos and conditioners, hair styling products and cosmetics include: BHT/BHA, parabens, petrolatum (and other petroleum-based substances), sodium lauryl sulfate and coal tar dyes. All of these have been proven to cause cancer and disrupt hormonal function. Some cause neurological and reproductive problems, and over time, with repeated use, can cause serious illness. Because the list of toxic ingredients in personal care products can be so extensive, we recommend consulting a book like Ruth Winter's *A Consumer's Dictionary of Cosmetic Ingredients, 7th Edition: Complete Information About the Harmful and Desirable Ingredients Found in Cosmetics and Cosmeceuticals* for more information on toxic substances to avoid.

Coconut or palm kernel oil is an excellent substitute for toxic, petroleum-based skin lotions. Petroleum-based products actually strip the skin of its natural oils, while coconut oil is very moisturizing to it.

A few cosmetic companies sell natural, mineral-based makeup products, which are safer for the body than conventional makeup. Most still contain a few toxic ingredients, but they are much better than other types of makeup. Natural makeup can be expensive, but so is cancer. Indeed, the results of one study, conducted by Berkeley's School of Public

Health at the University of California, revealed 32 brands of lipstick to contain cancer-causing heavy metals such as lead, cadmium and aluminum. The study concluded that prolonged use of lipstick could increase the risk for developing a variety of different cancers. And how many women use lipstick daily?

Antiperspirants also contain toxic heavy metals, particularly aluminum, which has been proven in studies to cause Alzheimer's dementia, Parkinson's and other neurological disorders. Antiperspirants also prevent the armpits from releasing toxins, so that those toxins continue circulating throughout the body instead of leaving it as they are supposed to do.

It's inconvenient to perspire, especially in public, but so is getting sick from your antiperspirant. Non-toxic deodorants don't stop perspiration but they do reduce its odor. Wearing loose-fitting clothing is one way to ensure that if you do perspire in excess, nobody will notice! In the end, the inconvenience of sweating must be weighed against the possibility of suffering brain damage or getting Alzheimer's down the road, or having toxins build up in your body because your antiperspirant is preventing their release. You could always keep the toxic stuff around for when you have an important business meeting or presentation, but only allow yourself to use it occasionally.

Health food stores sell natural deodorant, but you can also make your own with potato vodka and baking soda. You can also make your own perfumes using potato vodka and aromatic oils. Instructions on how to make various types of homemade deodorants and perfumes can be found on the Internet on many website blogs and health sites.

Coconut or palm kernel oil is an excellent substitute for toxic, petroleum-based skin lotions. Petroleum-based products actually strip the skin of its natural oils, while coconut oil is very moisturizing to it. Coconut oil also has innumerable health benefits, and we highly recommend reading Bruce Fife's *The Coconut Oil Miracle* to learn more about this amazing natural food. Polynesian and Hawaiian women have young-looking, healthy skin because they use coconut oil as a moisturizer. Even at 60, 70 and 80, many look half their age.

> I have found that most medical issues, even seemingly complex ones, like diabetes, depression and heart disease, can be successfully treated without the use of drugs.
>
> —Dr. Lee Cowden

PHARMACEUTICAL DRUGS—ARE THEY REALLY GOOD FOR US?

Pharmaceutical drugs are another major source of toxicity to the body. Yet most of us, whenever we hear the term "drug detox" don't think of physician-prescribed drugs as one of the toxins that we need to eliminate from our bodies. Instead, we envision a person with a cocaine or heroin addiction! We all know that street drugs harm the body, but many people are unaware that pharmaceutical drugs of all kinds are toxic to the body, too—the body treats them as harmful chemical substances that pollute it and impair its normal functioning.

The pharmaceutical industry has convinced most of us that medications heal the body, but consider this—no chemical substance that is found in pharmaceutical drugs is natural to the body, and the body was not created to handle these chemicals, so why would the body want it?

> **Most drugs benefit the pharmaceutical company, not the patient. They are good for the drug company's pocketbook, but not necessarily for you.**
>
> **—Dr. Lee Cowden**

At times, drugs can be used effectively to treat symptoms of illness, but they almost always damage the body in some manner and their chemical residue often remains in the body for years, long after you have finished taking them.

I have found that most medical issues, even seemingly complex ones, like diabetes, depression and heart disease, can be successfully treated without the use of drugs. This isn't common knowledge, however, as drug companies invest billions of dollars to convince people of the merits of pharmaceutical drugs, and pharmaceutical-company sponsored medical school professors don't teach their soon-to-become physicians about natural alternatives to [manufactured] drugs.

Occasionally, drugs are necessary for treating certain conditions and are useful in emergency situations, but they aren't good for the body when taken long term. In addition to damaging the body, they usually only mask symptoms and push whatever disease they are intended to treat even deeper into the body rather than fixing the underlying problem. Most drugs benefit the pharmaceutical company, not the patient. They are good for the drug company's pocketbook, but not necessarily for you.   —Dr. Lee Cowden

Statin drugs, for instance, which are used to lower blood cholesterol levels and are some of the most widely prescribed drugs, increase the risk of developing congestive heart failure and diabetes. According to Suzy Cohen, America's Pharmacist™ (*DearPharmacist.com*), the reason diabetes occurs is because statin drugs cause what is called "statin-induced hyperglycemia." This is not a true case of diabetes, but a condition caused by pancreatic damage and the death of beta cells that result from taking the drug.

Suzy contends, "When you pull the [statin] drug out of the picture, then the body's blood-sugar levels will start to come down. It's important to keep this in mind if you've been taking a statin and then suddenly develop 'diabetes.' That may, or may not, be the real diagnosis."

In addition, statin drugs suppress the production of Coenzyme-Q10 in the body. Co-Q10 is needed by the body, especially the heart, to produce energy, so people who take statins don't make enough Co-Q10 to keep their skeletal muscles, brain, heart muscles and other vital organs working well. The heart requires more Co-Q10 than any other organ because it makes more energy than any other organ. So people who are deficient in Co-Q10 are at a higher risk for developing congestive heart failure and arrhythmias (abnormal heart activity) and can even die from these side effects.

Finally, statins also suppress vitamin D levels, which the body needs to fight infection. Suzy Cohen says, "If you are on a statin drug and you cannot come off it, it's important to supplement the body with Co-Q10 and vitamin D to restore to the body what these 'drug muggers' are stealing from it."

Thus, statin drugs don't necessarily increase the quality or length of a person's life, and may even shorten it.

Other types of pharmaceutical drugs that are toxic and cause more harm than good are synthetic female hormones, which are often prescribed to peri-menopausal and menopausal women. These hormones increase the risk of breast, uterine and other types of cancer. The most commonly prescribed estrogen product in the United States is derived from the urine of pregnant horses. Several of the estrogens found in horses are not found in humans and actually cause further imbalances of estrogen in the human body. So why put these types of estrogen into humans when they are not naturally found in humans?

For more information about the toxic effects of different types of pharmaceutical medications and safe, non-toxic alternatives, we recommend that you visit The Academy of Comprehensive Integrative Medicine website: ACIMConnect.com.

Similarly, all progesterone-like drugs are made from chemicals called progestins, rather than from real hormones. These progestins only minimally resemble the human female hormone progesterone, which means that doctors are prescribing chemicals, not hormones, to replace deficiencies of natural hormones in women, and the body treats these chemicals as toxins.

Fortunately, compounding pharmacies have learned to create what are called bio-identical hormones, which are hormones that are chemically identical to what the human body makes. These bio-identical hormones are well received by the human body and do not increase cancer risk. When properly prescribed, bio-identical hormones cause all of the organs, including the detoxification organs, to work better, since optimal detoxification depends on good hormonal function, especially in older men and women.

Bio-identical hormones are a better solution for peri-menopausal and menopausal women than the synthetic drugs manufactured by pharmaceutical companies. Bio-identical progesterone is available over the counter without a prescription as a cream, which you rub into the skin. Most estrogen products, however, require a prescription.

Sadly, since drug companies lose money to the companies and compounding pharmacies that produce natural hormones, they are trying, through their influence with the U.S. Food and Drug Administration (FDA), to make compounded and natural hormones unavailable to the public. As a society, we need to protest stringent FDA regulation over compounding pharmacies and supplement companies so that in the future we don't lose our freedom to purchase natural remedies.

Anti-depressants, as well as sleep and anti-anxiety medications, are a third example of prescription drugs that are toxic to the body. And it goes without saying that street drugs are also toxic! All of these negatively impact the body's ability to make neuro-transmitters, which are important chemical messengers in the brain and body that regulate mood, energy and sleep, among other functions.

I have seen lots of people who have taken street drugs who are not the same after being on these drugs unless they detoxify them from their bodies.

Street drugs are fat-soluble chemicals that bind to fatty tissues in the body. Their breakdown products are continually released into the bloodstream from the fatty tissues over time, and cause symptoms.

Fortunately, if you have ever used street drugs or prescription anti-depressants or sleep medications, you can remove a lot of the chemical residue from the drugs from your body by doing infrared sauna therapy and oil pulling, and by taking certain types of toxin binders and/or homeopathic remedies. We describe these detoxification strategies later on in the book.

—Dr. Lee Cowden

Even if you have never taken prescription medications, it's good to do detoxification therapies, because chances are, you have some of the residue from these drugs in your body simply because the drinking water supplies of the largest U.S. cities contain fairly high levels of pharmaceutical and street drugs.

These drugs get into the drinking water when waste-water is treated with chlorine, then are dumped into a river or creek and subsequently taken up as drinking water by a city downstream. It may be difficult to believe that our drinking water supply is contaminated by drugs, but many studies and reports, such as the February 2009 *CBS News* report, "Probe: Pharmaceuticals in Drinking Water," have shown this to be true. The Philadelphia Water Department even admits on its website that the water supply contains pharmaceutical drug residue, but contends that the water is safe to drink. Yet how can water tainted with any amount of drug be safe? Read on to learn more about how to remove these contaminants from the body.

For more information about the toxic effects of different types of pharmaceutical medications and safe, non-toxic alternatives, we also recommend that you visit The Academy of Comprehensive Integrative Medicine website: *ACIMConnect.com.*

RADIOACTIVE ELEMENTS AND WAYS TO PROTECT YOUR BODY FROM THEM

So far, we've discussed how the body becomes toxic as a result of unhealthy food, water, personal care products and drugs, as well as what we can do to cleanse our bodies of them.

Unfortunately, our bodies aren't just affected by the toxins in things that we ingest or put on our skin. We're also affected by what we inhale, and one of the most dangerous inhalants to which we are all exposed daily is radiation—elements such as strontium, cesium, uranium, radium and plutonium.

One of the easiest ways to remove radioactive substances from the body is with zeolite supplements, which are minerals that come from volcanic rock. Iodine is beneficial for protecting the body against radiation damage.

Many of these are now prevalent in the environment because of the nuclear meltdown that occurred in Fukushima, Japan, in March 2011. When the tsunami that caused this accident damaged a nuclear power plant, radioactive elements were scattered over many miles. The Japanese government determined that the only reasonable way to deal with the radioactive waste generated by Fukushima was to burn it. So since the accident in 2011 they have been gradually burning its waste, and the radioactive elements from this waste are being dispersed across the globe. This radiation is contaminating our bodies and increasing our susceptibility to illnesses of all kinds, particularly cancer.

Fukushima isn't the sole cause of dangerous radiation in the environment, however. Other sources of harmful radiation exist. For instance, we now have radioactively powered satellites that are starting to fall out of orbit. Also, many types of warfare weaponry release copious amounts of radiation into the air.

All of these radioactive elements build up in the body and over time cause DNA damage that can lead to cancer. At some point in the near future, it is likely there will be a worldwide cancer epidemic because most people are unaware of the damage that radiation does to the body and don't know how to prevent it.

Like all toxins though, there are ways to minimize radioactive damage and the cancer risk that comes along with it. One of the easiest ways is with zeolite supplements, which are minerals that come from volcanic rock and are the best substances for removing radioactive elements from the body. NutraMedix is one company that makes two high-quality, homeopathically imprinted zeolite products that are excellent for this purpose.

Vitamin C also removes radioactive elements and heavy metals from the body. One of the best and longest-acting forms of vitamin C that is good for this purpose is Bio En'R-G'y C from Longevity Plus. This vitamin C product is most effective if taken daily, along with another product called Beyond Chelation (also made by Longevity Plus), which contains many beneficial nutrients that help the body detoxify a variety of environmental contaminants.

Iodine can also help to protect the body, particularly the thyroid, against radiation damage, since the body uptakes radioactive iodine from the air if we don't ingest sufficient levels of healthy, non-radioactive iodine.

Lugol's is one effective iodine solution that can help protect the thyroid from radiation, as well as support its function. Dr. Cowden has found liquid iodine to be a better choice than iodine tablets or capsules, as the latter two can get into the intestine (instead of being absorbed through the stomach) and damage beneficial bacteria there.

Finally, vitamin D3 protects against radioactive injury, as do the algae chlorella and spirulina. Washing vegetables in Chlorox diluted with lots of water also removes radioactive particles from food.

Taking one or more of these nutrients or products can greatly help to detoxify and protect your body against damage from radiation.

Toxic Foci in the Mouth/Dental Cavitations

People who are sick know that they have harmful microbes in their bodies—bacteria, viruses, parasites and so on—but did you know that most of us, whether sick or not, carry harmful bugs in our bodies? These microbes may or may not be causing disease and infection, but if so, it's important to eliminate them because they generate biotoxins and cause inflammation, both of which harm the body. While it is beyond the scope of this book to focus on detoxifying the body of all types of infection, we mention here a few common types of infection that may be causing us to feel less than our best.

First, it is common for people to have infection in what are called toxic foci. A toxic focus is an area in the body where there is a high concentration of disease-causing microbes (fungi, bacteria, viruses, etc.), biotoxins and manmade chemicals. Foci are created when some predisposing weakness or problem in a particular area of the body causes toxins and microbes to be attracted to that area.

Eighty percent of all toxic foci are located in the neck and head. The most common areas of infection are the tonsils, wisdom-tooth extraction and root canal sites, and the sinuses. Tooth-extraction sites are a popular place for toxic foci because most tooth sockets aren't properly cleansed and sanitized after the teeth have been removed. Indeed, many studies have shown that most root canal and extraction sites are infected, and these infections are often disseminated throughout the body and eventually cause disease in other parts of the body.

It is possible to remove teeth without causing infection in the jaw, but only certain types of dentists, called biological dentists, really understand how to do this. Hal Huggins, DDS, who was one of the first dentists to prove the dangers of root canals and dental amalgams, trained many dentists in proper tooth extraction and safe dentistry. The following website contains a list of these trained dentists:

HugginsAppliedHealing.com/find-dentist.php

In the United States, many pregnant women eat too many grains and not enough vegetables and fruits. They also don't take enough of the bio-available form of folate (methyl-folate), which results in children with small upper palates who don't have enough room in their mouths for their third molars (wisdom teeth). When this happens, in adolescence, the wisdom teeth have to be extracted, which then creates the potential for infection at the extraction sites.

> With the help of an Asian medical doctor, I created a nine-herb Chinese poultice that my patients could put into their mouths, using gauze pads. I discovered that this poultice resolved most of the infection in the mouth that had resulted from root canals and wisdom-teeth extractions.
>
> —Dr. Lee Cowden

If you have ever had a wisdom tooth extracted, or a root canal performed, there is a good chance that you have some infection in your mouth, even if you don't feel sick or have mouth pain. So it's usually a good idea to eliminate that infection to avoid getting sick down the road.

Toxic foci in the mouth, tonsils and sinuses can also create disease in other parts of the body, particularly the organs, in two different ways. First, the body has a system of energy pathways, called meridians, which start in the face and pass through every tooth and organ of the body.

So when a wisdom tooth site gets infected, for instance, the energy along that tooth's meridians gets disrupted and at the same time disrupts the functioning of the heart and small intestine, which are also found along those meridians. So a problem in a tooth can cause symptoms, weakening or disease in any other part of the body that's connected to the same meridian. Once an organ along a meridian becomes sufficiently weakened, it also starts to weaken the tooth that caused it to have problems in the first place, so eventually both the tooth and the organ weaken one another!

The Huggins Dental Network, as well as most competent biological dentists, can usually offer options for replacing infected root-canal teeth.

If you have had your wisdom teeth removed, it is essential to properly treat any infection in those bony cavitations (tooth-extraction sites), because any infection there can cause heart disease or problems in the digestive tract. I have successfully treated many heart disease patients by simply recommending that they go to a biological dentist to get their wisdom teeth cavitations cleaned out. —Dr. Lee Cowden

I used to think that having a root canal was no big deal, until I started hearing stories about people with severe illnesses, such as ALS and multiple sclerosis, who completely recovered once they had their root canals removed. I also personally know two people who were disabled by symptoms of chronic Lyme disease but who improved radically after they had their infected dental sockets cleaned out. —Connie

Root canals cause infection in the jaw, which later spreads to the entire body. The famous dentist, Weston Price, DDS, established this fact in the 1920s, through his meticulous experiments on rabbits.

Years ago, whenever patients would come to me with root-canal issues, I would tell them that these teeth had to be removed since they were causing jaw infection. This mandate was not popular among my patients, so I came up with a more practical approach for eliminating jaw infections.

With the help of an Asian medical doctor, I created a nine-herb Chinese poultice that my patients could put into their mouths, using gauze pads. I discovered that this poultice resolved most of the infection in the mouth that had resulted from the root canals and wisdom teeth extractions. For many patients, the poultice would enable them to avoid dental surgeries to remove infection. Often, however, the root canal infections would resolve but then recur, because the infection was in the dental tubules of a tooth and there was no way to sterilize the tubules of that tooth.

So now I teach other doctors to tell their patients that if a chronically infected tooth or jaw area isn't yet causing a life-threatening disease, they don't have to get it surgically treated. Instead, they can use the Chinese poultice, then wait and watch to see what happens over time. If at some point the infection starts to cause a serious disease, then the patient needs to get it surgically cleaned out immediately.

So far, that approach has worked pretty well. It's now rare for patients who are treated that way to get a life-threatening disease from a root canal or infected cavitation, as long as 1) they are checked twice yearly by a biological dentist or health care practitioner who can perform special types of testing to see what organs that tooth site might be affecting, and 2) they use the nine-herb poultice that I developed and recommend.

—Dr. Lee Cowden

If you do have to get a root-canal tooth removed, options exist for replacing that tooth, such as a dental bridge or removable partial denture, although such alternatives aren't without their own problems. For this reason, some people choose to do nothing to replace the tooth. However, the Huggins Dental Network, as well as most competent biological dentists, can usually offer options for replacing infected root-canal teeth.

Another way to kill bacteria in the mouth and discourage the development of foci infections there is by doing a treatment called "swish n' spit" with hydrogen peroxide. We won't be outlining that procedure here, but we encourage you to visit the ACIM website (*ACIMConnect.com*) for step-by-step instructions.

DENTAL AMALGAMS: A MAJOR SOURCE OF TOXICITY

Foci infections aren't the only toxin problem that many of us have in our mouths. Dental amalgams, which are comprised mostly of mercury, are also extremely toxic to the body. Over time, these amalgams leech mercury into the brain and body, and cause or contribute to the development of neurological illnesses such as Alzheimer's dementia, Parkinson's and multiple sclerosis. They also cause immune suppression and a variety of metabolic problems.

Dental amalgams can be easily replaced with a plastic composite material, but the amalgams must be removed by a holistic or biological dentist who understands the dangers of improper amalgam removal.

For more information on the dangers of dental amalgams, we highly recommend reading the book *Amalgam Illness: Diagnosis and Treatment* by Andrew Hall Cutler, PhD, which can be found at: *NoAmalgam.com*.

If you have dental amalgams, it's important to get them removed, if you can afford it financially. Even if you don't have an immediate toxic reaction from the metals in your dental work, at some point you could develop an allergy to them, which would then cause an autoimmune reaction throughout your body. The MELISA Medica Association (*melisa.org*) does blood tests to identify heavy-metal sensitivities.

Metallic and porcelain crowns are also toxic. Porcelain crowns are usually made of stainless steel beneath the porcelain, which means that they contain nickel alloys. When you eat an acidic food, it etches the nickel out of the stainless steel and you then end up swallowing and becoming allergic to that metal.

Dental amalgams can be easily replaced with a plastic composite material, but the amalgams must be removed by a holistic or biological dentist who understands the dangers of improper amalgam removal, and the importance of taking special precautions in their removal. It is unwise to allow just any dentist to remove your amalgams. Improper removal of amalgams can cause greater amounts of mercury to be disseminated throughout the body, and can cause immediate damage and illness to the body. You can get a referral for a good biological dentist through Hal Huggins' website: *HugginsAppliedHealing.com*.

Cleansing/Detoxifying the Sinuses

Sinus problems or foci infections in the sinuses are another common source of toxicity to the body. We breathe in lots of "critters" that get into our sinuses and produce toxins. These toxins end up poisoning the bloodstream, then the organs and other tissues of the body. These infections can also cause heart and blood vessel problems because when the sinuses drain, they affect the tonsils, which then affect the heart and circulation meridians of the body. So it's important to eliminate lingering sinus infections.

Now, just because you aren't blowing your nose ten times a day or not sniffling, doesn't mean that you don't have a sinus infection that's affecting your immune system and body. Many people have some degree of infection in their sinuses, so even if you have no obvious symptoms, it's best to assume that an infection could be present and periodically cleanse your sinuses with saline and aloe vera. Even if you don't have a sinus infection, whenever you irrigate your sinuses with saline you are flushing out poisonous toxins that could be adding to the toxic burden of your body.

A good rule of thumb is to irrigate the sinuses daily for one to four weeks (depending on the amount of infection present) and then monthly after that.

Sinus irrigation can be accomplished by using a Neti pot, or piston or bulb syringe. This is a simple procedure, but if you want to make sure that you do it right, step-by-step instructions about how to irrigate the sinuses can be found on the ACIM website: *ACIMConnect.com.*

When irrigating the sinuses, you usually begin with one cup of warm saline. It's important to make the saline the correct strength and temperature. Most people use too much salt and burn their nose and sinuses. The proper dosage can be achieved by mixing one-fourth of a teaspoon of salt in a cup of tepid or warm water. Typically, one cup of water will be sufficient to irrigate both sides of the nose, unless you use a Neti pot, in which case you might need two cups because it's not as efficient as a bulb or piston syringe.

After a week of irrigation with just saline, you can then add a little less than half a tablespoon of whole-leaf filtered aloe vera to the cup of saline. Aloe vera is a potent antimicrobial remedy and will help to remove any stubborn infection that remains in the sinuses. If pathogens are present, it can produce a burn-ing sensation in the sinuses, especially the first time that you irrigate them with aloe.

After irrigating once daily for a while, the sinuses eventually become healthy enough so that bugs don't want to live there anymore and the burning sensation with the aloe will no longer occur. A good rule of thumb is to irrigate the sinuses daily for one to four weeks (depending on the amount of infection present) and then monthly after that.

> In 1990, I discovered that most acute sinus bacterial infections were really caused by an underlying chronic fungal infection. When I treated my patients with anti-fungal herbal remedies, they never had bacterial sinusitis again. About ten years later, the rest of the medical community also discovered this fact.
>
> I also found that I could clear up my patients' chronic fungal infections with an oral herbal remedy by NutraMedix called Banderol, along with an herb called Pau D'Arco, and by putting them on a low-starch, no-sugar and no-fruit diet for eight weeks. If they did this at the same time that they irrigated their sinuses daily, the chronic infections usually resolved.   —Dr. Lee Cowden

GOOD ALL-AROUND STRATEGIES FOR TOXIN REMOVAL

Juicing

Vegetable juicing is an excellent, inexpensive way to cleanse the body of some of the environmental and food toxins that we've mentioned thus far. When we consume no food other than freshly juiced vegetables, our bodies start to spontaneously detoxify. Also, the body uses about a third of its energy to digest food, so when you drink juice instead of eating solid food your body can direct some of the energy that it would otherwise use for digestion to heal, detoxify and rebuild the body.

Vegetables also contain large amounts of nutrients that your body needs to function properly. These nutrients become more available and usable to your body when it receives them in liquid form. When the body expends large amounts of energy to process solid food, as noted above, if you have any problems in your gastrointestinal (GI) tract, some of that food may end up getting discarded instead of used by the body.

Some vegetables and fruits are especially beneficial for detoxifying the organs. Parsley, watermelon, pineapple and celery, for instance, detoxify the kidneys. Dandelion greens detoxify the liver.

Also, some undigested foods can get fermented or putrefied by microbes in the gut, and the putrefied by-products will then be absorbed through the intestines into the blood vessels that lead to the liver. This creates toxicity in the liver and subsequently in the other major organs of the body. Juice fasting thus allows the liver to detoxify itself because it is not being overloaded by undigested, putrefied solid food each day.

Similarly, water fasts assist the healing of the body by cleansing the cells and giving the organs a chance to rest and repair themselves. When the GI tract, liver, kidneys, pancreas and other organs don't have to expend energy to process and metabolize food for energy, this allows them to heal. Unfortunately, water fasts are difficult for many people, so a vegetable juice fast may be a better option for most.

Some people like to do a juice fast using fresh fruit. While it may be okay to include some fruit in a juice fast, fruit tends to cause fungal overgrowth in the gut, especially in people with compromised immune systems or health problems. Most people today have fungal overgrowth, due to the abundance of sugar and antibiotics in our food supply and the toxins in our environment.

If you know that you have fungal overgrowth in your gut, juicing root vegetables such as carrots and beets may not be a good idea, either, since they tend to have a lot of natural sugar in them, which can also feed fungus. Of course, carrots and beets contain vital nutrients for cleansing and healing the body, particularly the liver and lymphatic system, so some people may be able to include them in their juice fasts. If you choose to juice carrots and beets and/or other root vegetables, it's best to use only organic vegetables, since non-organic root vegetables are full of pesticides and the goal of a fast is to take toxins out of the body, not put more back in!

> Harmful emotions are often stored in the liver and gallbladder. Because of this, it's beneficial to consider doing an exercise called Visualization Raging prior to a liver and gallbladder flush. This exercise enables the body, particularly the detoxification organs, to release any harmful emotions that might be stored there.

Sometimes, it's a good idea to combine fasting for health reasons with fasting for spiritual reasons. When you get toxins out of your body, it's amazing how much easier it is to think and hear from God. If you are unaccustomed to fasting, start with a one-day fast first. If you can tolerate that, you can then increase to a longer fast over time. Immediately following the fast, don't eat a fatty, heavy meal like pizza, as your gallbladder may become inflamed and you may experience severe abdominal discomfort. Instead, slowly add fats and protein back into your diet in small amounts.

Some vegetables and fruits are especially beneficial for detoxifying the organs. Parsley, watermelon, pineapple and celery, for instance, detoxify the kidneys. Dandelion greens detoxify the liver. If you don't like dandelion greens, then juice the leafy green tops of beets, which also remove toxins from the liver.

LIVER/GALLBLADDER FLUSHES

Over the years, environmental toxins accumulate in the liver and gallbladder, creating a build-up of gallstones and/or biliary sludge in the gallbladder and bile ducts, which then drain toxins from the liver into the intestines for clearance by the body. When enough of these stones, sludge and toxins build up, the bile fluid cannot drain into the intestines and the liver cannot clear other toxins from the body. Normally, the liver sends toxins through the bile ducts into the intestines for clearance by the body, but some of these toxins remain in the liver if it is overloaded. Over time the liver becomes increasingly toxic and incapable of performing its job of toxin removal.

Also, anger and other painful unexpressed emotions can contribute to liver and gallbladder toxicity and disease. Many healthcare practitioners in the United States and elsewhere have discovered that these emotions aren't just stored in the brain, but also in other organs and tissues of the body. Over the past several centuries, Chinese health practitioners have observed that one of the reasons why people develop gallbladder disease is because of unresolved, accumulated anger and frustration that builds up inside of the liver, bile ducts and gallbladder.

For about five days prior to the flush, it's essential to increase your intake of vitamin C, fiber and magnesium.

What's more, stored emotions in the liver, bile ducts and gallbladder can contribute to an accumulation of physical toxins in those areas. Environmental toxins and pathogenic microbes often congregate in regions of the body where toxic emotions and emotional trauma are stored. When these emotions get released, the body more readily releases and removes the environmental toxins and microbes.

Because of this, it's beneficial to consider doing an exercise called Visualization Raging prior to a liver and gallbladder flush. This exercise enables the body, particularly the detoxification organs, to release any harmful emotions that might be stored there.

To do Visualization Raging, find someplace in your home where you won't be heard by other family members or your neighbors, such as a walk-in closet in the bedroom. Alternatively, go out into the countryside. Then picture the faces of all the people who have frustrated, hurt or angered you throughout your life, and imagine them as if they were there with you. Then yell at them, one by one, for all the things that they said or did that hurt you, or for all the things that they failed to say or do that hurt you.

Start with your past acquaintances and distant relatives, then move to your close family members, and finish up with God and yourself. When you shout at yourself, stand in front of a mirror, if possible, and visualize yourself at several previous ages. Then shout at yourself for all the things you did or failed to do at those ages. After you have released all of the pent-up anger towards your family, friends, God and self, forgive yourself, God and every person at whom you shouted.

After you do Visualization Raging, you can then go on to do the liver/gallbladder flush. For this, you'll want to first soften any stones that might be in the gallbladder or bile ducts. This is important because the flush will cause the gallbladder and bile ducts to contract very strongly. If you have hard stones in your gallbladder, then those stones can get pushed into the common bile duct and ultimately cause secretions from your pancreas to back up and remain in the pancreas. When this happens, you can end up in the hospital for pancreatitis and have to get any trapped stones surgically removed from the bile ducts!

Fortunately, this scenario can easily be avoided by taking a tablespoon of apple cider vinegar three times daily or fifteen drops of orthophosphoric acid (OPA) for five days prior to the flush. The only company that sells OPA is Progressive Laboratories in Irving, Texas. When you take OPA, make sure that you put it in a little bit of water, drink it quickly, then take another drink of water, and swish it around inside of your mouth, because OPA can etch the enamel off the teeth. OPA is also useful for melting kidney stones.

For about five days prior to the flush, it's also essential to increase your intake of vitamin C, fiber and magnesium. These nutrients help the body to clear the bowels so that when the bile stones and bile sludge get dumped into the intestine they don't get re-absorbed back into the body through the intestinal lining but are instead moved out of the body. Ideally, you want to have at least one or two bowel movements daily.

You might start with 1,000 mg of vitamin C and 100 mg of magnesium twice daily, then slowly increase the amount of each until you get one or more loose bowel movements per day. Then, add fiber to the mix to get the bowel movements more formed again.

Certain foods, such as cow dairy products and gluten grains, as well as fungus and parasites, tend to clog the lymphatic system. So if you want to keep your lymphatic system functioning optimally, it's also important to consume as little gluten and dairy as possible and treat the body for these infections.

Important: People with kidney failure should not take high doses of magnesium since this could cause fatal cardiac or respiratory arrest. Also, people who have what's called a G6PD deficiency shouldn't take vitamin C. G6PD deficiency is a rare but serious condition in which the body cannot properly process vitamin C due to a missing enzyme.

If you take a low dose of vitamin C, such as 500 mg, and have fatigue, pink urine or otherwise feel sick, it may not be a good idea to increase your vitamin C dosage as these can be indicators of the enzyme deficiency. If you suspect that you have this deficiency because you have a negative reaction to vitamin C, a simple blood test for G6PD enzyme can verify whether or not the deficiency is present. Most people, however, can take supplemental vitamin C without a problem, so unless you have never taken a vitamin C product in dosages above 500 mg, there is probably no need for concern.

At bedtime on the day of the flush, take a large dose of magnesium citrate or another high-quality type of magnesium, along with the highest dose of vitamin C achieved during the build-up period. Then drink two ounces (1/4 cup) of olive oil or another healthy oil, such as walnut or almond oil. Chase that down with 1/4 cup of lemon juice. Then go to bed immediately after that and lie on your side.

> I prefer to lie on my left side, since the gallbladder duct is best positioned to release stones on this side. In reality, it's okay to lie on either side, but don't lie on your back. If you fall asleep and end up on your back before morning, that's fine, but at least try to fall asleep on your side, since most of the gallbladder contraction to release stones will happen within the first hour or so after you go to sleep. —Dr. Lee Cowden

Lymphatic Drainage

To maximize the benefits of this flush, it's also a good idea
to stimulate and cleanse the lymphatic system the day before
and the day after the flush. The lymphatic system is part of the
circulatory system, comprising a network of tiny vessels that
carry toxins out and away from the tissues and organs. These
toxins are dissolved in a clear fluid called lymph, which is
dumped into the bloodstream near the heart and then cleared
from the bloodstream either by the kidneys or liver. If the
lymph fluid is flowing well, especially in the abdominal lymph
vessels, then the lymph vessels in the liver and gallbladder can
more easily drain other toxins away from those organs.

One of the easiest ways to stimulate the movement of lymph
and toxins through the lymphatic system is by using a lymphatic
drainage machine, which can be purchased on various Internet sites
for less than $100. Chi Machine International (*ChiMachine4u.com*)
sells what are called Chi devices, which are more expensive
lymphatic devices.

These devices gently move the body from side to side in a
fishlike movement. This causes a rhythmic passive contraction
of the muscles surrounding the lymph vessels and stimulates
the movement of stuck toxic lymph fluid so that it is more easily
shuttled out of the body. To use the machine, you simply place
your ankles in a cradle that sits atop the machine while lying on
your back on the floor. The motorized device then moves the
ankles and body side to side while you relax.

Bouncing up and down on a rebounder, or mini-trampoline, for five to ten minutes is another way to stimulate the drainage of toxins from the lymphatic system. Rebounders also exercise the body and oxygenate the tissues. If you can't afford a high-quality rebounder, which costs around $300, jump-roping or pretend jump-roping provides a similar effect.

Perhaps the simplest and cheapest way to stimulate the lymphatic system is to pretend bike-pedal on the floor or bed. This involves lying on your back and raising your legs up in the air, and then moving them in a circular bike pedal motion for five to ten minutes. You can rest periodically as needed while doing the exercise.

Finally, certain foods, such as cow dairy products and gluten grains, as well as fungus and parasites, tend to clog the lymphatic system. So if you want to keep your lymphatic system functioning optimally, it's also important to consume as little dairy and gluten as possible and treat the body for these infections.

Saunas, Biomats and Clay Plaster Treatments

Juicing and gallbladder flushes are two important ways to get toxins out of the body. But there are other therapies you may also want to implement to help your body eliminate the more deeply entrenched and embedded toxins. Saunas are one of the most important of these.

Many years ago, I had a 57-year-old patient who suffered from neuropathy. This condition caused him not to be able to feel anything but a pins-and-needles sensation below his knees. I tested him for diabetes and vitamin B-12 deficiency, since both of these conditions can cause neuropathy.

He had neither, so I told him that he probably had some toxins in his body, although I didn't know what kind. I suggested that he do sauna therapy, because it would possibly rid him of whatever was causing the neuropathy.

Far-infrared saunas mobilize toxins from deep within the cells and cause the body to release them through the sweat. They heat the body from deep within its core, unlike gym saunas, which mobilize fewer toxins.

So the man took my advice, and went to a sauna to detoxify his body. When he did, the whole sauna became saturated with the smell of gasoline! The other people in the sauna had to leave because the smell was so strong. The man had never been exposed to gasoline on a regular basis before, except for one summer when he was seventeen-years-old and had a job washing carburetor parts in gasoline with his bare hands. He had carried gasoline in his body since that time, for about 40 years, and all the while it had been damaging his nerves, until it finally created symptoms in his body.

After he regularly did sauna therapy for a while, the neuropathy vanished, without him having to do any other therapy.

This story illustrates just how powerful and important sauna therapy can be for removing toxins, especially far-infrared saunas, which are very effective for removing environmental toxins of all types. Far-infrared saunas mobilize toxins from deep within the cells and cause the body to release them through the sweat. They heat the body from deep within its core, unlike gym saunas, which, while beneficial, don't mobilize as many toxins.

Initially, sauna therapy can be done for 10 to 45 minutes per session, about every two to three days. Some people can build up to doing one to two sessions per day, but if you have chronic fatigue or get easily depleted and tired from exercise or stress, you may not be able to do more than one or two sauna sessions per week. I recommend starting off with 15-minute sessions and building up to 45-minute sessions. Start at 100 to 110°F and build up to 145 to 150°F.   —Dr. Lee Cowden

Another way to remove toxins from the body is with a Biomat. This is a little mat that you lie on which heats up. It stimulates detoxification by increasing the flow of oxygenated blood throughout the body, but it can also be used as an ideal alternative to a sauna, especially for those who don't have large enough rooms in their homes to set up a regular sauna.

Another way to maximize the benefits of sauna therapy is to put a tablespoon of olive oil or other type of healthy oil into your mouth during the last three to five minutes of the sauna, and then swish it around.

To create a sauna from the Biomat, start by rolling out the Biomat on the bed or the floor. Then, place two layers of terry cloth bath towels on top of it, so that you don't damage it with your sweat. Lie down naked on top of those towels, and place another towel and a couple of old blankets on top of yourself, so that you get nice and hot. You can leave your head uncovered so that you don't feel as hot but you will still be mobilizing a lot of toxins from their storage sites in the body as if you were in a sauna.

New saunas usually cost $2,000 or more, although used two-person wood saunas can sometimes be found on the Internet on places like eBay or Craigslist for less than $1,000. A new Biomat may cost about $1,500. If you don't have the money for either of these, a third way to do a sauna-like treatment is to heat your bathroom as high as possible with an electric heater and then sit in that room until you sweat.

To maximize the effect of a sauna, you can rub some moistened clay mud all over your bare body while heating up the bathroom or your wood sauna. Clay pulls toxins from the body and binds them so that they stick to the clay, rather than getting re-absorbed and re-circulated throughout the body. French green clay and bentonite clay, which you can purchase at health food stores and on the Internet, work well for this purpose. If you do clay therapy, it's important to cover only part of your body the first time you do a sauna —say, your arms or legs—to avoid mobilizing too many toxins at once. You can get sick from excessive toxin release if you cover your entire body with clay the first time around. You can incrementally increase the amount of clay that you use each time you do a sauna.

Whichever sauna or sauna-like method you use, it's important to shower with glycerin soap immediately following your sweat session so that the mobilized toxins that are on the surface of your skin don't go back into your body.

Another way to maximize the benefits of sauna therapy is to put a tablespoon of olive oil or other type of healthy oil into your mouth during the last three to five minutes of the sauna, and then swish it around. Whatever toxins were mobilized by the sauna and are floating around in your bloodstream will be pulled through the lining of your mouth and bound by the oil that's in your mouth. After swishing the oil around for several minutes, you can then spit it out into a flushing toilet or running sink. This technique is called "oil pulling."

All of the body's blood passes through the mouth at least once per minute, so if you keep some oil in there for at least three minutes, you can bind a significant amount of the toxins that are in the bloodstream. It's also beneficial to do oil pulling first thing in the morning, since the body heats up during the night and mobilizes toxins, some of which are still floating around in the bloodstream when you awaken.

If you do oil pulling in the morning, it's a good idea to pour the tablespoon of oil into a small glass at bedtime the night prior to the treatment and set it at your bedside so that you don't have to get up in the morning to get the oil. This is important because the body cools when you get out of bed and pushes the mobilized toxins back into the cells. Oil pulling is the cheapest method that we know of for removing fat-soluble toxins from the body, so we highly recommend giving it a try.

Toxin Binders

Physical therapies for removing toxins, such as juicing, saunas, rebounding and Chi machines, while important, aren't always sufficient for removing a lifetime of accumulated toxins from the body.

To get the most out of any detoxification program and ensure that you're getting all difficult-to-remove toxins such as heavy metals, radioactive elements and others out of the body, it's also essential to take oral toxin binders on an ongoing basis. The amount and type of toxin binders that you need depends upon your overall state of health and the particular health problems that you may have.

Heavy metals are a very harmful type of toxin that must be removed from the body. This can be accomplished using special toxin binders called EDTA, DMSA and DMPS, which are powerful chemical substances that can be taken either orally or intravenously, under physician supervision.

There are many types of toxin binders on the market, but not all of them remove all types of toxins. For instance, two products—EDTA and DMSA—are specifically designed to remove heavy metals, while cholestyramine and some fiber products are beneficial for removing mycotoxins produced by fungi. (The topic of mold and fungi will be covered in Part Two of this book, *Create a Toxin-Free Home*). For the purposes of this book, we will only be mentioning a few of the best and most common toxin binders and their uses and benefits.

The body is continually bombarded with a variety of industrial contaminants, some of which have already been described in this book. Common toxin binders that are useful for removing many of these environmental contaminants include: chlorella (and other algae), glutathione, modified apple and citrus pectin, and zeolite. These binders are usually safe to take long-term as part of a comprehensive wellness plan that focuses not only upon removing toxins from the body, but also keeping it clean so that new toxins don't build up there. Consider taking one, two or even three of these binders on a daily, ongoing basis for these purposes.

Of particular importance are heavy-metal toxin binders. All of us are exposed to heavy metals in the environment, which are prevalent in our food supply (especially fish), water and air, as well as in dental amalgams and vaccines. Heavy metals accumulate in the body and over time cause severe neurological and immune system damage, and disrupt the functioning of nearly every system and organ in the body.

Neurological diseases such as multiple sclerosis, autism, Parkinson's and Alzheimer's disease are thought to be caused, at least in part, by heavy metal toxins, as are many autoimmune and chronic health conditions such as chronic fatigue syndrome and fibromyalgia. Indeed, many studies support these hypotheses. Metals also impair many metabolic processes and interfere with the body's ability to remove other types of toxins. Heavy metals are, therefore, a very harmful type of toxin that must be removed from the body. This can be accomplished using special toxin binders called EDTA, DMSA and DMPS, which are powerful chemical substances that can be taken either orally or intra- venously, under physician supervision.

Unlike other types of detoxification therapy, it's not a good idea to do heavy metal removal on your own. It's important to work with a healthcare practitioner who thoroughly understands heavy metal chelation—or detoxification—therapy, since improper dosing of heavy metal binders can cause metal toxins to be redistributed throughout the body, instead of removed from the body.

Laser Energetic Detoxification (LED), is a rapid, gentle, and non-invasive method for removing chemicals, heavy metals, sulfa drug residue and food/chemical sensitivities from the body.

Taking the wrong binders or in the wrong amounts can also cause the body to become overloaded and sick as a result of having to process too many toxins all at once. Intravenous chelation, especially, carries significant risks and should only be done by a holistic physician who specializes in heavy metal removal.

Heavy metal removal can take years, as metals accumulate deep within the body's organs and tissues, but with time, as the body's metal load is reduced, you will be surprised at how much better you will feel as a result of having done this type of detoxi- fication. Therefore, it's essential to consider heavy metal toxin removal as part of your daily cleansing regimen.

Homeopathy

Homeopathy is another important type of medicine that can be used in different ways to detoxify the body. All toxins are comprised of measurable energetic frequencies, which can be captured and transferred into a prepared remedy; for instance, into a vial of liquid. The frequencies in that vial can then be applied to the body, to remove whatever toxin is contained within the vial, such as the energetic signature of a heavy metal toxin. This principle of "like curing like" is known as homeopathy. That is, a substance that causes symptoms in large doses can be used in tiny amounts (as in the energetic signature of a toxin) to treat those same symptoms.

> I have developed an innovative detoxification strategy that combines homeopathy with light therapy. It's called Laser Energetic Detoxification (LED), and is a rapid, gentle, and non-invasive method for removing chemicals, heavy metals, sulfa drug residue and food/chemical sensitivities from the body.
>
> For LED, I use a special technology to imprint the energetic frequencies of different toxic chemical substances and allergenic foods into a glass vial containing a liquid remedy of some type. I then take a laser or infrared light and pass it through the vial, and sweep that light over the body in a specific fashion. The light effectively transfers the energetic information from the vial into the body and stimulates the body to remove whatever toxins are contained within the vial.
>
> LED is based upon homeopathy, quantum physics, and detoxi-fication principles. Usually, homeopathic remedies are taken

under the tongue as pellets or liquid drops. However, for LED, light is used to deliver the homeopathic remedy to the body.

Before I do an LED session, I assess the patient for chemical toxins through muscle testing (Applied Kinesiology) or via an electrodermal screening system such as the Zyto. These tests can assess the body for the presence of sulfur-based compounds, chemical toxins, heavy metals and other toxins that may be affecting them.

One LED session can often remove more toxins from the body than several months of oral detoxification therapy, and when done periodically, patients recover from chronic conditions much more quickly. For more information about LED, and practitioners that use this kind of therapy, visit the Academy of Comprehensive Integrative Medicine website: *ACIMConnect.com*.

—Dr. Lee Cowden

Homeopathic drainage remedies are another type of homeopathic treatment, designed to significantly support the body's natural detoxification processes. They are especially important to use during the initial phases of detoxification, when you are trying to eliminate lots of contaminants from your body, or when you are sick and have compromised organ function.

These remedies strengthen the detoxification organs—particularly the liver, kidneys and lymphatic system—and cause them to be more efficient and effective at removing toxins. Pekana and Heel make excellent homeopathic remedies, and NutraMedix makes herbal products that have homeopathic-like effects upon the body. Some particularly excellent products from NutraMedix include: Burbur Detox, Parsley Detox, Pinella Brain and Nerve Cleanse, Sparga, Zeolite and Zeolite-HP.

Also, nutritional supplements such as creatine monohydrate, molybdenum, zinc, tri-methyl-glycine, 5-methyl-tetrahydro-folate (a special type of folic acid that is easily absorbed and used by the body), along with vitamins B-6 and B-12, can help the body process and remove toxins, especially in people with sub-optimal genetics, compromised immune systems and/or compromised liver function.

Part Two

Create a Toxin-Free Home

In Part One we described a few common toxins that are making many of us sluggish, tired, irritable or just downright sick, as well as solutions for removing these from the body. Yet many other sources and types of toxins exist, many of which come from our home and work environments. These toxins represent more of the "dirty-water faucets" that we need to turn off so that our proverbial bathtubs aren't continually being filled with more murky water.

> **The cleaner your home is, the better your health will be, regardless of your current health condition.**

To do this, it's essential that we de-contaminate the places where we spend the most time. We must do this before we can effectively remove these household toxins from our bodies. In the following sections, we describe some common household toxins and how to remove them from the home and/or workplace, as well as the body.

Again, some of us may be able to get away with remediating only a few aspects of our environment, while others will want to implement most, if not all, of the suggestions we offer in this part of the book. The more health problems you have, the more changes you may need to make to your living and work environment in order to be successful in your wellness journey. This is because the fewer the burdens that your immune system has to deal with, the better it can help you to heal. At the same time, the cleaner your home is, the better your health will be, regardless of your current health condition. We realize that most people can't do everything we suggest, and therefore we recommend doing only what you can, and what's most essential, so that you don't get discouraged because you can't do everything perfectly!

Toxins in the Home

Nearly all homes contain toxins that can seriously affect the health of your body and mind. It's easy for most of us to accept that outdoor air is polluted, but did you know that, according to the Environmental Protection Agency website, the air inside most homes is, on average, five times as polluted as outside air? But research studies show that indoor air can be as little as three times more toxic, or as much as fifteen times more toxic, than the air outside! Even if the home is located in the most polluted city in the United States, the air outside is still cleaner than the air inside, with few exceptions.

Most of us like to consider our homes as a place of refuge, where we can rest and recover from the world. But if our homes are loaded with toxins, then an environment that is meant for rest and recovery can actually become a war zone for the body, whether we realize it or not.

So why are our homes so toxic? Find out why in the following sections, and what you can do about it.

HOUSEHOLD CLEANING PRODUCTS

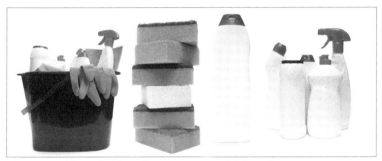

Commercial household products contain multiple toxins.

Most of us wouldn't drink our household cleaning products because we know they would make us sick. But did you know that every product that comes into contact with your skin, or which you inhale, goes into your bloodstream and then into your tissues, as if you had eaten it anyway? So don't breathe in or clean your furniture, clothes, floors or appliances with anything that you wouldn't eat!

Besides the fact that most household cleaning products will make you sick to your stomach if you swallow them, they also contain chemicals that have been proven to cause cancer, allergies, neurological problems and hormonal dysfunction, among other health issues.

Therefore, removing these toxic products from the home is essential for healing or simply staying well and ensuring that your tissues don't get loaded with lots of cancer and disease-causing "junk." So the first step to take is to throw out your chemically-laden household products and purchase instead eco-friendly products that are made entirely of natural ingredients.

How do you know if a product is toxic to your body? Well, as a general rule, cleaning products are toxic if they have a strong chemical smell or ingredients that you can't pronounce or which you have never heard of before. Conventional supermarkets carry a few non-toxic household products, but such products are found in greater abundance and more often at better prices in health food stores.

Start by replacing your laundry detergent, dishwasher soap and other household cleaning products, such as sink, toilet, cabinet and floor cleansers, with natural products such as those made by Seventh Generation or Planet, Inc. This goes for any building, repair or gardening materials, such as pesticides, paint, adhesives, and laminating substances.

Carpeting and Flooring

The United States is one of the few nations in the world that uses carpet throughout its homes. Unfortunately, carpeting is a major cause of dirty, toxic air. Most carpets are synthetic and contain formaldehyde (the same chemical as embalming fluid!), a potent toxin that causes asthma, allergies and cancer, and which continually outgases into the air and pollutes it. Remember

doing frog dissection workshops in middle school? And
that potent, stinky smell that came from the frogs that made
you nauseated? Well, that smell was formaldehyde, and it
was what was used to preserve the frogs so that they wouldn't
decompose. That's the same
chemical substance found in the
carpeting of most U.S. homes.

**These days it's possible to
purchase hardwood floors that
snap together and which don't
require glue to adhere to the
surface of the sub-floor. This,
or terrazzo tile with non-toxic
grout, are the least toxic types
of flooring material.**

Carpets also contain
chemicals such as DDT and
other pesticides, as well as dust,
bacteria and fungi, which aerosolize into the air, get into the
lungs and harm the body in a
variety of ways. Most carpets also have carpet padding beneath
them, which is also loaded with that frog-preserving, toxic
formaldehyde.

In addition, the adhesives that attach some types of flooring
to the sub-floor beneath it are toxic. Such adhesives outgas
benzene, toluene, hexane and other solvents, which can cause
susceptible people to develop dizziness, confusion, brain swell-
ing, heart rhythm disturbances, lung inflammation, immune
suppression and other problems.

These adhesives are used in the glue to make it liquid so that
it can be easily spread across the floor. Rarely do we attribute
carpeting and other toxic flooring to the reason why we might
feel less than optimal some days, or downright sick, but carpet
and floor toxins can add a burden to the body that, along with
other toxins, over time causes symptoms and illness.

Of course, not everyone is susceptible to sickness from carpeting, but if you have a compromised immune system or already suffer from a serious health condition, you may be. If you fall into this category, you may want to consider moving or replacing the carpeting in your home with hardwood or tiled flooring, especially in the bedroom.

If you can afford it and are able, though, no matter your health condition, we recommend exchanging your carpeting for hardwood flooring throughout your home so that your air and body will be cleaner.

These days it's possible to purchase hardwood floors that snap together and which don't require glue to adhere to the surface of the sub-floor. This or terrazzo tile with non-toxic grout are the least toxic types of flooring material. Many homes in Europe and South America are hardwood, and they promote a cleaner, fresher environment than carpet. When choosing a hardwood floor, it's important to avoid those that are painted with polyurethane or other toxic substances, unless they are baked on to the surface of the material. Pure wood is most ideal. Once you have the wood snapped or nailed down, you can protect the surface against scratches and stains by coating it with tung oil, which soaks into the wood.

Tile is another fairly non-toxic option for flooring but the space between tiles is filled with grout, and some grout is toxic. So if you plan to use tile, it's best to use non-toxic grout, which can also be sealed with tung oil. Even then, it's important to periodically clean the grout thoroughly (such as with a toothbrush), because toxins from the air can accumulate there. Therefore, unless you like to get down on your hands and knees to scrub the floor, hardwood flooring may be a better option than tile.

Concrete is also a decent replacement for carpet, although concrete can be hard on the joints and cause back and knee pain in people who are susceptible to pain. Concrete flooring can be purchased in a variety of textures and colors, and fashioned to look like brick, tile and other types of flooring. Concrete can also be painted, to keep it from becoming porous, but it's important to use low-VOC (volatile organic carbon) paint, which is less toxic to the body than other types of paint. Most large paint companies now make low- or no-VOC paints.

Finally, another reason why it's better to have a hardwood, tile or concrete floor is because carpets require vacuuming. Vacuuming is problematic because vacuums pick up chemicals and dust and throw them into the air. When you breathe in that air, your lungs then become a filter for the chemicals and dust, and your lungs and body then get filled with the same garbage that you see in the vacuum bag!

A recent study conducted by the EPA revealed that homes in certain geographic areas of the northeastern United States contained high levels of DDT because people were bringing it into their homes on the soles of their shoes.

For people that live in cold climates and who want warm or soft floors in the winter, it's okay to put washable throw rugs on top of the hardwood flooring, since these rugs can be tossed into a washing machine and cleaned regularly to remove any toxins or dust.

Again, we realize that it's not realistic or feasible for everyone to remove the carpeting in their homes, but if you know that you are strongly affected by environmental chemicals, or are already sick with a chronic health condition, you may want to consider replacing the carpet in your home with one of the safer floor options that we mention in this section, or else consider moving to a home with better flooring.

Furniture and Window Coverings

Believe it or not, some furniture can also be a source of harmful household toxins, especially pressed-board furniture, which is filled with formaldehyde (yes, that embalming agent again), solvents and other chemicals that we have already described. If you look beneath your furniture and see that it looks something like sawdust pressed together, consider exchanging it for solid wood, because that pack-board—or sawdust-like wood—contains formaldehyde.

One easy way to reduce the amount of toxins in the air in your home is to use vertical blinds or pull-down shades rather than curtains. Curtains attract chemical and microbe-containing dust, so every time you shake them or take them down, you also shake chemicals and dust loose, which then gets into your lungs. Vertical blinds are better than horizontal ones because dust settles more on horizontal blinds than vertical ones.

Purchasing pull-down shades for the bedroom is also a good idea, since shades can create a blackout effect in the room at night. This is important because studies have shown that during bright moonlit nights, people don't sleep as well as a result of the moonlight coming in through the window. The body responds to that light and the pineal gland in the brain stops producing adequate amounts of melatonin, which is critical for deep, restful sleep. So getting better sleep is another side benefit of pull-down shades.

The Problem with Wearing Shoes in the Home

Asian cultures had a good idea when they created the custom of taking their shoes off at the door. Shoes can bring pesticides and other chemical toxins into the house, which then get into the body and increase the risk for developing allergies, hormonal problems and occasionally even serious illnesses such as cancer and neurological disease.

Most of us don't think much about wearing shoes inside our homes, but we would never put our shoes on the kitchen countertop! But if you wouldn't contaminate your countertop with dog poop or chemical fertilizers, why would you pollute your carpet with these things? Especially since the pollutants don't just stay on the carpet, but get aerosolized into the air you breathe.

DDT, a once commonly used pesticide that is now banned in the United States because it was proven to cause cancer, is an especially toxic substance to drag into the home. Even though DDT is no longer used in the States, a recent study conducted by the EPA revealed that homes in certain geographic areas of the northeastern United States contained high levels of DDT because people were bringing it into their homes on the soles of their shoes.

So even though DDT is no longer used in the United States, the half-life of DDT in grass is up to fifty years, which means that a large part of what was sprayed on the grass in years past is still in the soil and some of us are stepping into that soil and tracking DDT into our homes. That DDT then gets into the carpet and air of the home, and we end up breathing it.

The Pesticide Action Network (*PANNA.org*) describes some of the harmful effects of DDT on its website. They note that the pesticide has been associated with liver, breast and pancreatic cancer (among other types of cancer); male infertility, miscarriages, early menopause, birth defects and motor skill problems. In children, it has been associated with a decrease in verbal, memory and other perceptual performance skills.

If you have tracked a bit of DDT or other pesticides into your home, it's unlikely that the levels will be high enough to cause disease, but there may be enough of the chemical present to adversely affect your immune system and add to the toxic burden of your cells. So it may be worthwhile to consider leaving your shoes at the door, especially if you already have health problems or compromised immune system function.

Fortunately, it's easy to remove this source of toxicity from the home by simply having two sets of shoes—one for indoor wear and another for outdoor wear. By switching your outdoor shoes at the main entryway with your indoor shoes, you can prevent toxic chemicals from the lawn, sidewalk and air outside from getting into your house.

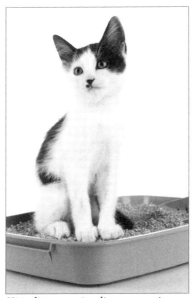

Kitty litter carries disease-causing toxins.

PET TOXINS

We love animals but we have to admit, keeping a cat litter box inside the main living area of your house isn't the best idea if you want to keep your body as healthy and toxin-free as possible. Cats often carry a bacterial infection called leptospirosis, as well as a parasitic infection called toxoplasmosis. Both toxoplasmosis and leptospirosis can be transmitted through kitty litter and can cause serious illness that is difficult to treat and recover from.

These microbes can be aerosolized into the air every time your cat scratches in the litter box, and breathed in by anyone who happens to be nearby. While it's unlikely that you will contract either of these infections just because you own a cat, if you have a compromised immune system or serious illness you may want to consider setting aside a special room for your cat's litter box, and not spend too much time in that room. It's also a good idea to have a special set of shoes for wearing in the cat room, because litter tends to get on the floor, and you don't want that litter in the rest of the house.

Finally, if you create a special room for your cat's litter box, consider purchasing a separate air conditioning or heating unit for that room also, rather than keeping the central air conditioning or heating ducts open, since the toxins from the kitty litter/animal waste can be transmitted through the ducts, into the rest of the house.

Owning a dog, while healing to the soul, can also present challenges to wellness, especially in people who already have significant health issues. Dogs often carry parasite eggs and cysts and other disease organisms from the outdoors into the house, so you may want to consider restricting your dog's access to certain parts of the house.

In the colder months, the most effective way to clean the air is with a high-efficiency purification of air (HEPA) filter or similar high-quality air purification product. Austin Air and Nikken make high-quality air filters. These filters have fine pores and charcoal, which pull most dirt, animal dander, carpet chemicals, paint solvents and other contaminants from the air.

For instance, it may not be a good idea to let your dog sleep in bed with you. One of the advantages to owning a dog over a cat, though, is that dogs go outside to relieve themselves, and therefore don't aerosolize into the air all of the microbes that are in their bodies, as so happens when cats use a litter box.

Of course, being able to do such things as cuddle, sleep with and pet your cat or dog can be very healing, especially if you live alone and the pet is a deep source of companionship and joy. For this reason, you'll want to weigh the pros and cons of our suggestions and decide whether, given your living and health situation, it's practical and feasible for you to make these changes.

If you're really sick and/or indifferent about whether your cats and dogs spend most of their time outdoors, you may decide it's best to keep them mostly as outdoor pets or, if the weather is cold, to confine them to certain parts of the house.

On the other hand, if you aren't struggling with severe health issues, or your pet is like family to you, you might find that the stress or sadness of having to confine your dog or cat to certain parts of the home suppresses your immune system more than the toxins or parasites that the animal might bring into the home. So it's up to you and your doctor to decide upon a situation that would be best for you and your animals.

Cleaning the Air Inside Your Home

As previously mentioned, the air inside most homes is full of toxins from chemicals in the carpet, furniture and flooring. Wall paint, cleaning supplies and other chemical substances, such as air fresheners, also contribute to toxic air in the home. As these toxins build up in the body, they cause allergies, which can lead to autoimmune disease and a myriad of chronic health conditions—even cancer.

I have seen some people become seriously ill as a result of simply having used air fresheners for a couple of months!

> Fortunately, these toxins can be removed and illness easily
> avoided by removing these substances from the environment.
>
> —Dr. Lee Cowden

After you've eliminated all toxic substances from your home, the easiest and cheapest way to eliminate toxins from the air in the warmer seasons is to open two windows on opposite sides of the house and run a fan in one of those windows, so that it blows toxins out the window on one side of the house and sucks clean air into the house through a window on the other side of the house. You can cut the amount of air toxins in half just by doing this for a couple of hours daily.

If your finances are limited, owning plants is another fantastic way to remove toxins from the air.

In the colder months, the most effective way to clean the air is with a high-efficiency purification of air (HEPA) filter or similar high-quality air purification product. Austin Air and Nikken make high-quality air filters. These filters have fine pores and charcoal, which pull most dirt, animal dander, carpet chemicals, paint solvents and other contaminants from the air.

Owning a HEPA or other type of high-quality air purification filter is a great way to ensure that your lungs won't take in all of the garbage from your home environment! Because these filters emit electromagnetic fields, which can disrupt sleep, it's best to run them in the bedroom during the daytime, when you aren't sleeping and your body isn't regenerating. If you can only afford one filter for your home, you might run that filter in the bedroom(s) during the day and then in the living room, kitchen or family room at night.

Another way to make sure that you're breathing in the cleanest air possible and not inhaling massive amounts of contaminants is to change your HVAC (heating, ventilation and air conditioning system) filters often. If you can find filters that have charcoal in them, in addition to fiber, then this charcoal will bind some of the chemical toxins that are in the air. These filters are called activated carbon air filters and are more expensive and not as readily available in stores as traditional HVAC filters, but you can purchase them on the Internet.

One way to eliminate microbes (such as mold spores, which will be discussed later in this book) from the air in your home is with aromatic oil and a steam humidifier. Simply place a few drops of aromatic oil into a small humidifier, which you can purchase at Target or Wal-Mart, and fill the humidifier with water. Certain aromatic oils have antimicrobial properties, and when they are diffused into the air via a humidifier they can kill and remove harmful microbes in the air. Thieves' oil, which is available on the Internet, is particularly potent. Some essential oils, such as rosemary, eucalyptus, lemon, cinnamon, thyme, oregano and tea tree oil, are also good and leave a pleasant aroma in the environment.

If your finances are limited, plants are another fantastic way to remove toxins from the air. Certain plants work better for this purpose than others. Philodendrons and certain types of ivy, for example, absorb chemicals from the air—everything from formaldehyde and hexane to benzene, xylene and toluene, and others.

Toxins in the Garage

Finally, it's also a good idea to eliminate any toxic chemicals from your garage if possible, especially if you leave your car in there. This is because any chemicals from the garage can also get into your car so that every time you get into your car, you breathe in those aerosolized chemicals. The best way to store any toxic chemicals that you may require for outdoor projects is in a separate, detached storage unit or shed.

Electromagnetic Radiation (EMR)

Electromagnetic radiation (EMR) is a generally under-appreciated, but extremely dangerous toxin that is found in nearly every home today. In the following sections, we describe EMR, its sources and effects upon the body, and how to remove it from the home.

But before we do that, we want to share a story that illustrates the damaging effects that this toxin can have upon human health.

Numerous studies show that the current levels of EMR to which most of us are exposed daily damage the body, and over time, can commonly cause fatal illnesses such as cancer. These reports have been published in the scientific- and medical community-supported BioInitiative Report (*bioInitiative.org*).

Around 1990, a man and his wife came into my office for a routine wellness exam. After doing a series of conventional medical tests on them, I discovered that they both had cancer. I was perplexed, because they were only in their early 40s and seemed to be happy with their lives. Neither had ever been exposed to extreme levels of toxins.

I then suspected that there might be dangerous electromagnetic radiation in their home and that this was what had caused them to develop cancer. So I sent a building biologist (someone who specializes in EMR detection and remediation) to their home to measure the EMR with an electromagnetic field meter. The biologist discovered that the fields over the couple's bed were 100 times above U.S. government standards (and most building biologists consider the U.S. government's standards to be extremely lax as it is!).

So the husband unplugged their clock radios on either side of the bed, as well as the television at the foot of the bed, and by just doing these things the electromagnetic radiation levels came down to normal. The couple left their three bedroom appliances unplugged for two months, and when they came back to see me two months later, their cancers had completely vanished without any other therapy. I monitored them for four more years and they remained healthy. So they both had had cancers that were caused principally by electromagnetic radiation.

—Dr. Lee Cowden

This story is just one of many proving the potential dangers of excessive exposure to electromagnetic radiation (EMR). It is an insidious yet invisible toxin that needs to be removed as much as possible from our bodies and homes, if we want to heal from our current chronic health conditions or simply feel our best. If you have a serious health condition or illness, you may even find it impossible to completely recover until you remove the EMR from your environment.

Electromagnetic radiation is emitted from all kinds of sources—ranging from Wi-Fi and cell phones to appliances, telecommunications towers and power lines. It cannot be seen and is usually not felt by the person at the time of exposure. Many people therefore mistakenly assume that it isn't harmful, and evidence about its damaging effects upon the body hasn't been widely published in mainstream media.

The U.S. government has also set extremely high limits for EMR exposure that far exceed what scientists who don't profit from EMR industries deem to be safe. For all of these reasons, people are falsely led to believe that this type of toxin isn't a big deal.

EMR has been linked to cancer, autoimmune and other diseases, and, along with mold, is probably the most dangerous toxin in most homes today.

The telecommunications industry has also convinced people through its advertising that owning smartphones, cordless phones and Wi-Fi-enabled devices are a necessary and normal part of life. Exponential advances in the development of ever-more-attractive technological products make it difficult for people to turn down these products because they make their work and personal lives more productive, efficient and financially profitable. The benefits of technology make it incredibly difficult for people to say "No" to their dangers.

Yet numerous studies show that the current levels of EMR to which most of us are exposed daily damage the body, and over time, can commonly cause fatal illnesses such as cancer. These reports have been published in the scientific- and medical community-supported BioInitiative Report (*BioInitiative.org*), as well as other medical journals. The BioInitiative Report is compiled by an international working group of scientists, researchers and public health policy professionals who have conducted more than 2,000 studies on the damaging effects of EMR.

Magda Havas, PhD, at Trent University in Canada, has produced an excellent 24-minute YouTube video called "Wi-Fi in Schools is Safe. True or False?" that provides compelling proof about how Wi-Fi and other sources of electromagnetic radiation harm the body.

> Interestingly, whenever I talk to health-conscious people about the importance of eating organic food, avoiding chemical contaminants and drinking clean water, most will agree with me. Yet when I talk to these same people about the importance of detoxifying the home of excessive electromagnetic radiation, they will look at me sideways or debate about how we need Wi-Fi and smartphones to survive in today's world. —Connie

Yet EMR has been linked to cancer, autoimmune and other diseases, and, along with mold, is probably the most dangerous toxin in most homes today. Even if it doesn't make you sick right away, it will make you sluggish and alter your body's biochemical processes. These processes are driven first and foremost by energy, and the negative energy that comes from EMR disrupts the body's natural energy so that its systems cannot function properly.

In a May 2000 interview, the late orthopedic surgeon and Nobel Prize nominee Robert Becker, MD, who is also widely known as "the father of electromedicine" and author of *The Body Electric* and *Cross Currents*, stated, "I have no doubt in my mind that, at the present time, the greatest polluting element in the earth's environment is the proliferation of electromagnetic fields."

Today, one in two people is developing cancer. According to studies, some of these cancers have been linked largely, or in part, to EMR exposure. This means that as EMR levels continue to increase, the incidence of cancer and other diseases caused by EMR are likely to increase as well.

The amount of EMR in the environment is increasing exponentially every year as new telecommunication towers are constructed, Wi-Fi replaces hard-wired Internet connections, fluorescent light bulbs replace incandescent light bulbs, and so on. We don't mean to be negative, but the truth is, we are constructing for ourselves an incredibly dangerous environment in which to live.

In some Western European countries such as Switzerland, Austria, Germany and Denmark, electromagnetic pollution is more widely recognized and accepted as a health hazard. According to information taken from a chart in the award-winning book,

Wireless Radiation Rescue, by Kerry Crofton, PhD, safety standards for EMR exposure are much stricter in those countries. According to Dr. Crofton, even Russia and China have stricter standards for EMR exposure than the United States.

In addition to creating cell mutations and damaging DNA (DNA gives our body the genetic instructions for how to develop and function), electromagnetic pollution in the home negatively impacts immune function. It disrupts the normal functioning of the neurological, cardiovascular and hormonal systems by altering inter- and intra-communication among cells. As if that weren't enough, it disrupts the functioning of the blood-brain barrier, which separates the blood in the body from the brain's fluid. This barrier helps to keep toxins out of the brain, so any such disruption allows damaging toxins to easily enter the brain.

Cell phones cause brain damage, and many brain cancers have been linked to cell phone usage.

Many scientists and researchers have established and confirmed these findings. For instance, Dr. Crofton, in her book, *Wireless Radiation Rescue,* notes that Professor Cherry discovered that EMR confuses and damages the cells' signaling system and in some cases, as with cell phone use, nearly drowns out the signals. Disruptions in cell signaling, Cherry learned, produces symptoms such as headaches, concentration difficulties, memory loss, dizziness and nausea, and long-term diseases such as Alzheimer's dementia, brain tumors and depression. Other scientists and researchers, including those who have contributed to the Bio-Initiative Report, have confirmed the above-mentioned findings.

Solutions for Reducing EMR

So what are the most dangerous sources of electromagnetic pollution in the home and what can we do to eliminate them so that our homes aren't a war zone of radiation but instead peaceful, cell-friendly environments?

Well, first, if you have Wi-Fi Internet, it's better to replace it with a hard-wired broadband connection. Having a wireless Wi-Fi router is like having a mini-antenna inside the home. According to Stan Hartman, environmental consultant for RadSafe in Boulder, Colorado, when people have Wi-Fi antennas inside a router on their desks, they are getting about the same amount of radiation as if they were 30 meters (90 feet) or less away from the large outdoor antennas of a typical cell phone base station (though the Wi-Fi signal typically isn't as constant as a cell phone signal).

To put that into perspective, scientist Roger Santini found that people who live within 300 meters (about 900 feet) of a cell phone tower have a much greater incidence of a variety of health problems—including fatigue, irritability, headaches, nausea, anorexia, insomnia, depression, brain fog and cardio-vascular disease, as well as many other health issues—than those who live further away.

Another way to lower EMR in the home is to exchange all of your cordless phones for the old-fashioned corded ones. It's nice to be able to walk around your home and do things while talking on a cordless phone, but did you know that these phones emit constant radiation that is just as strong as that which comes from cell phones? DECT (Digitally Enhanced Communications Technology) phones are particularly dangerous. Also, cordless-phone base stations emit EMR and cause harm whether or not the phone is in use, so it's best to keep a corded phone in your home if you don't want to be exposed to constant, high amounts of radiation from cordless ones.

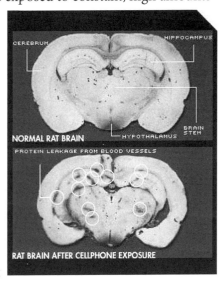

The top image represents the cross-section of a normal rat's brain and the lower image represents the cross-section of that same rat brain after a single two-hour exposure to cell phone radiation. This was from a study conducted by scientist Leif Salford: *TheTruth seeker.co.uk/?p=1808*. The dark spots in the lower image represent protein leakage from damaged blood vessels, indicating significant damage to neurons (part of the brain tissue).

As the above images and many studies illustrate, cell phones also cause brain damage, and many brain cancers have been linked to cell phone usage. Studies have also shown that when you talk on a cell phone, your red blood cells clump together and can't effectively deliver oxygen and nutrients to the other cells of the body.

Therefore, it's best to use your cell phone infrequently; for short calls only, and keep it turned off or in "airplane mode" while at home. Get a landline and encourage your friends and family to call you on that instead! If it's impossible for you to do this—because you need a cell phone for work, for example— use the speaker-phone option on the phone and keep it as far away from your body as possible.

Some people may benefit from sleeping on an Earthing sheet. This is a metallic-lined sheet (usually carbon- or silver-lined) that helps to normalize the body's energy and which may partially protect it from EMR.

One way to protect your body from EMR at night is with a Faraday cage, which is a metallic-lined mesh cloth net that drapes over a canopy bed or which is suspended from the ceiling and completely encloses the bed and shields out 99 percent of all high-frequency EMR from the bed while you sleep. High-frequency EMR comes from your neighbors' and your Wi-Fi; utility company smart meters, cell phone towers and other sources of microwave and radio frequency radiation. Since the body repairs itself during sleep, it's especially important to eliminate EMR at night. Owning a Faraday cage is especially important if you live in an apartment, condominium or townhome and have neighbors above, beneath and directly adjacent to you, each with his/her own Wi-Fi network and cordless phone.

Some people may also benefit from sleeping on an Earthing sheet. This is a metallic-lined sheet (usually carbon- or silver-lined) that helps to normalize the body's energy and which may partially protect it from EMR. This sheet is connected to a metal grounding cord, which is plugged into the round opening below the two vertical prongs on an electrical outlet or connected directly into the ground via a copper wire attached to a grounding rod. Electrons from the earth get transferred through the grounding wire to the sheet, and subsequently, to the body. These electrons elinimate free radicals that lead to DNA damage and cancer, and balance the body's energy and protect it so that it is less impacted by harmful EMR.

According to a study that was published in the June 2005 edition of the *British Medical Journal,* researchers found that children who lived within 650 feet of a power line had a 70 percent greater risk for developing leukemia than children who lived 2,000 feet away or more.

In some cases, it is best to use both an Earthing sheet and a Faraday cage in the home, but in other cases, one or the other will suffice. For more information about Earthing, visit: *EarthingInstitute.net.*

If you live in a multi-family dwelling, you may want to consider using a Faraday cage instead of an Earthing sheet, since there is some evidence that the sheets won't work well and may even be dangerous if there is a source of EMR above the bed, such as from the neighbors above you. If you purchase a Faraday cage, though, it's important to keep in mind that if there is a source of EMR beneath the bed (such as from the Wi-Fi of the people living below you), then the cage should completely enclose the bed. Fortunately, the companies that sell Faraday cages often also sell silver-lined fabric mesh that can be placed beneath the bed, so that the bed can be completely enclosed with the metallic cloth mesh.

In addition to Earthing sheets, the Earthing Institute also sells Earthing mats for your feet and Earthing wrist straps. These can be used to shield the body from EMR while you are sitting at your computer, since computers are another dangerous source of radiation. Laptops that are left plugged in and charging while you use them, are especially harmful—therefore, it's best to operate your laptop on battery power whenever possible, and never use the laptop on your lap.

Power Lines

The following suggestion for reducing EMR is radical, but sometimes life-saving. If you live in close proximity to major power lines, you may want to consider moving.

According to a study that was published in the June 2005 edition of the *British Medical Journal*, researchers found that children who lived within 650 feet of a power line had a 70 percent greater risk for developing leukemia than children who lived 2,000 feet away or more. Scientists who study EMR believe that high-voltage power lines should not be constructed anywhere near to where people work or live.

If you discover that your home is within range of dangerous EMR from power lines or another source and you aren't able to move, consider painting all of your walls and doors with EMR shielding paint and covering the windows with metal screening or shielding fabric. Before painting your walls, however, it's best to consult with an EMR expert to make sure you do it properly, as improper shielding can create more problems than it solves. More information about these shielding products and how to use them can be found at The EMF Safety SuperStore:

LessEMF.com/paint.html

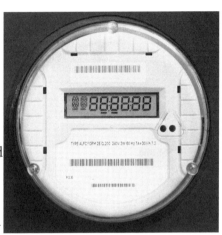

SMART METERS

Many U.S. homes, as well as some homes in Western Europe and Canada, now have smart meters installed on them. These are electrical meters that record electrical energy consumption at regular intervals throughout the day. The

Smart meters are a newer, but also very dangerous source of radiation toxicity in the home.

meters then relay that information back to the utility company for monitoring and billing purposes.

Many people oppose smart meters because they have increased energy costs for some and allowed utility companies to conduct indirect surveillance upon the homes of the people who have them. Most importantly, however, smart meters emit dangerous levels of cancer-causing radiation.

> I can testify firsthand to the health hazards of smart meters. When one was installed on my home, within a very short period of time I became fatigued and brain-fogged and developed atrial fibrillation (a potentially dangerous heart rhythm disturbance).

> I am exceptionally healthy, so the fact that the meter affected
> my well-being proves just how dangerous they can be, because
> a person with an illness or health condition would have likely
> suffered even more severe effects upon his/her health. Fortunately,
> once I was able to get the meter removed, my energy returned
> and other symptoms disappeared.   —Dr. Lee Cowden

Some states have created legislation that allows consumers to refuse smart meters if they don't want them installed on their homes. To learn more about the steps that you can take to refuse a smart meter on your home, or get one removed, we recommend visiting: *StopSmartMeters.org.*

If you live in a state that doesn't yet have legislation against smart meters or you don't have access to an organization that can help you to get yours removed, you may want to consider securing your analog meter behind lock and key (so that the utility company installers cannot replace it) and/or writing a certified letter to your utilities company refusing your consent to have a meter installed.

If a meter has already been installed on your home, revoke your consent of the meter via a certified letter to the utilities company and insist that they remove the smart meter by a specified deadline. Refuse to take "No" for an answer! It is your property, your body, and your well-being. An excellent documentary released on September 5, 2013, "Take Back Your Power," describes in greater detail the dangers of smart meters. To learn more, visit: *TakeBackYourPower.net.*

Home Appliances

Appliances in the home can be another problematic source of EMR. Getting rid of your microwave and limiting the use of other high-level radiation appliances isn't a bad idea, especially for people who know they are EMR-sensitive.

Microwaves are especially dangerous. You wouldn't put your head into a microwave, yet by standing outside one while it's cooking your food, you are exposing your body and brain to high levels of cancer-causing radiation. Microwaves also damage the nutrients in foods, which is another good reason to not have one.

Also, consider eliminating fluorescent light bulbs from your home. Besides being another major source of radiation, these bulbs cause mercury to be released into the environment whenever they are broken. LED (light-emitting diode) or incandescent bulbs are a better choice. Incandescent bulbs can still be purchased on the Internet. Even though LED bulbs are more expensive than incandescent or fluorescent bulbs, they use less power than traditional bulbs and last much longer, and so are more economical over the long run than incandescent bulbs or fluorescent bulbs.

Consider purchasing Graham-Stetzer filters, or Memon transformers, which greatly reduce the amount of radiation generated by electrical appliances and wiring in the walls and/or ceiling of your home or office.

Finally, the simplest and possibly most important way to reduce EMR in the home is to unplug all appliances in the bedroom at night, so that the body can regenerate and heal without the interference of harmful electrical fields from these appliances. In some cases, it's also necessary to turn off the electric circuit breakers in the breaker-box of the home before bedtime, so that your body isn't exposed to EMR from the home's electrical wiring.

A cheap way to measure the fields from electrical appliances/ wiring in the home is with a $35 Gauss meter, which can be purchased at: *LessEMF.com*. If the Gauss meter reads greater than 0.2 milligauss over your bed when the circuit breakers are on, then you should also turn off the circuit breakers at night. Yes, it can be a bit of a hassle to do this, but you'll get better sleep if you do, and your body will heal much faster from any chronic health conditions.

Finally, consider purchasing Graham-Stetzer filters, or Memon transformers, which greatly reduce the amount of radiation generated by electrical appliances and wiring in the walls and/or ceiling of your home or office. Electrical wiring in the walls radiates dangerous EMR several feet into the room, even when all of the electricity and electrical devices are turned off. For more information on these filters/transformers, visit: *StetzerElectric.com* or *MemonYourHarmony.com.*

> The Memon products may be superior to the Graham-Stetzer filters because they are also thought to shield the home against high-frequency electromagnetic radiation from outside sources such as Wi-Fi and microwave towers, not just the lower-frequency radiation from wall wiring and appliances. I own a Memon transformer and it has significantly reduced the amount of EMR in my home.   —Connie

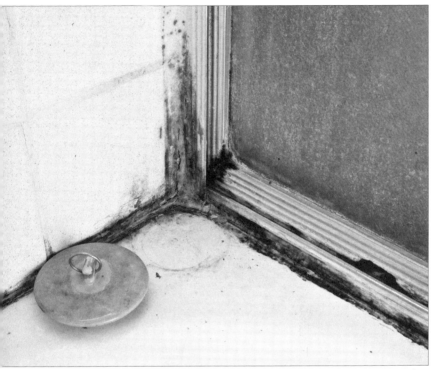

If any toxin could compete with electromagnetic radiation for the prize of most dangerous household toxin, mold would be it!

THE DANGERS OF MOLD

Mold is prevalent in many homes, yet many people don't realize that their walls, floors and ceilings are harboring this often colorful and fuzzy, at other times invisible, yet harmful toxin. And though it hides in the walls, it continually releases harmful spores and mycotoxins (toxic chemicals produced by molds) into the air we breathe, so that we end up getting sick from inhaling these spores and toxins.

One study of 10,000 U.S. homes, the results of which were published in *USA Weekend* in 1999, revealed more than 50 percent of these homes had levels of mold sufficient to cause health problems.

Mold specialist Ritchie Shoemaker, MD, writes in his book, *Mold Warriors*, that 25 percent of the population cannot effectively detoxify mold once they are exposed to it. This means that in such people, mold and its mycotoxins build up in the body over time and cause allergy symptoms and/or disease. These toxins may cause one person to feel a bit more sluggish than usual, while another may become bedridden with illness from them.

Fortunately, mold toxins can be removed, with a combination of homeopathic detoxification remedies, sauna therapy, and specific toxin binders and medications such as cholestyramine.

Even people who are able to detoxify mold from their bodies will often have red, itchy eyes, sneezing, allergies, fatigue or other symptoms for as long as they remain in a moldy environment. And just because the home doesn't smell musty or you can't see mold, doesn't mean that it's not present!

The mycotoxins produced by mold are more toxic and harmful to the body than any other manmade toxin except for some radioactive elements. They suppress the immune system and cause cancer, chronic fatigue and depression, among other illnesses, and predispose the body to a variety of autoimmune diseases. Mold toxins are also fat-soluble, which means that they get trapped in the body's fat tissues and accumulate there. Once in the body, they are very difficult to remove.

Fortunately, mold toxins can be removed, with a combination of homeopathic detoxification remedies, sauna therapy, and specific toxin binders and medications such as cholestyramine, which we discuss in greater depth in later sections of this book. Still, it takes time to get rid of them and the process can be laborious and complicated, especially if you are one of the 25 percent that doesn't automatically eliminate such toxins from your body.

Like most toxins, not everyone will react negatively to mold, especially if it's not present at high concentrations inside your home, but some will, so it's a good idea to eliminate it, if you find it lurking in your shower, sink, walls or other places inside your home or workplace.

Testing Your Home for Mold

So how do you know if you have mold? Well, if you find moisture or a leak somewhere indoors, chances are, mold or other fungi are present there. In order to get rid of that mold, you must first fix the water leak, or else any remnant of mold that remains alive after remediating the area will multiply and re-grow.

You may have a leak beneath a bathroom sink or around the shower, for instance; or around a toilet, dishwasher, clothes washer, ice-maker or bathtub. Examine every potential location in your home and feel around that area with your hands. If you feel coldness, it means that there is moisture there, even if you can't see the water. Assume it's a good idea to get rid of that source of moisture so that no fungi can develop there and wreak havoc upon your body.

In addition to visually checking for mold, you can order a do-it-yourself ERMI test. ERMI stands for "Environmental Relative Moldiness Index," and measures the presence and concentrations of more than 36 mold species in the home, based on a sample of dust. The ERMI test was developed by scientists at the Environmental Protection Agency. Home-testing kits can be obtained on the Internet at: *ERMIMoldTest.com.*

If you can't afford an ERMI test, which typically costs around a couple of hundred dollars, there is another do-it-yourself way to test for mold in your home.

First, obtain several culture dishes designed for growing fungi. These can be purchased in the plumbing department at Home Depot and some other hardware stores. Purchase a dish for each of the major rooms of your house. Be sure to put one in the washing machine room and one on a shaded windowsill outside.

Remove the lids and leave the dishes in their respective locations for an hour. Then pick up the dishes in the same order in which you opened them up so that the air-exposure time totals the same for each. Replace the lids and label the location of each plate on the bottom of the dish so that you can identify the rooms that the mold is in. Place all of the culture plates somewhere in your house away from direct sunlight for three days, since sun kills mold and fungus. Then, check the plates daily for colonies of fungal growth.

If any of the plates from inside the house has more colonies on it than the plate that was on the outside windowsill, then this means that there is a mold problem inside the house. The plates with the most amount of mold on them indicate the rooms with the greatest mold toxicity.

Having mold in your home, in and of itself, doesn't mean that your body is being harmed by it. However, if ERMI or culture-plate testing reveals that mold is present, and you also suffer from undiagnosed symptoms and are not feeling well, it is worth doing further testing to find out whether mold toxins are the cause.

Some molds and funguses, such as stachybotrys and some aspergillus species, are fairly deadly at low concentrations. Aspergillus niger, and the two most common species of stachybotryrs, are black. When it comes to fungus, black is bad! So if you see black fungus, you'll want to make sure to get it removed.

Mold Remediation

After you fix all of the leaks and sources of ongoing water damage in your home and have identified the areas where mold is present, remediate the affected area by spraying or cleaning it with a non-toxic substance such as vinegar, ozonated water or hydrogen peroxide.

If you find areas of drywall or flooring that have been water damaged, then that material must be replaced with brand new material. Otherwise, you will continue to breathe in mold toxins on an ongoing basis.

In places where the water damage has been extensive, you may need to call a professional mold remediator to remove the mold, but bear in mind that all mold remediation companies use toxic chemical fungicides to remove mold. However, if mold is extensively present, being temporarily exposed to some chemicals is probably the lesser of two evils, especially if you can leave your home for a while after the remediation and open the windows. This will allow some of the chemicals to dissipate into the air. If you have a charcoal HEPA filter, it's also good to run that after the remediation process.

If your home has been badly flooded by a hurricane (like those homes affected by Hurricane Katrina) you might as well plow that home down and rebuild it, since it can cost more than $40,000 to remediate mold and fungus in that kind of situation.

Ozone air purifiers are sometimes a good option for removing mold. They also remove some chemicals from the environment and will kill any disease-carrying mites, fleas or ticks that might also be present there. If you are going to use an ozone air purifier, though, don't use it whenever people, animals or plants are present in the room, because ozone can be harmful if you inhale it. It's a free radical that damages the body's cell membranes, the most critical of which are located in the brain. Therefore, it's best to leave the home and then open some windows after you are finished ozonating, to remove any traces of ozone in the environment.

Purchasing an ozone device with a timer on it is especially useful, so that any ozone that's produced has time to clear the environment before you return home. After a few hours, all of the ozone and harmful nitrates that are in the air will break down and dissipate. Make sure also to find a temporary place for your pets and plants to stay while you are ozonating the environment—perhaps with a friend or trusted neighbor.

It's also a good idea to periodically ozonate your car, especially the air conditioning system, as this is a prime location for mold spores to grow. Nearly all cars have mold in them, because they are continually exposed to moisture, both inside and outside.

Testing for Mold and Mycotoxins in the Body

Mold expert Ritchie Shoemaker, MD, developed an on-line test that you can do in front of your computer at home to check for mold toxins in your body. It's called the Visual Contrast Sensitivity test, costs just fifteen dollars, and can provide you with a first clue about whether your body is harboring mold and mycotoxins. The website where this test can be found is: *SurvivingMold.com.*

Mold and other fungi cannot be successfully removed from the body as long as you are consuming foods that contain sugar or starch. This includes all grains, legumes, starchy veggies (such as potatoes), fruits, fruit juices, alcoholic beverages and vinegar, as well as most dairy products.

If you fail the test, it means that there is a high likelihood that you have been exposed to mycotoxins, either recently or sometime in the past—even years ago—and that those toxins are now causing you health problems.

You may not have obvious symptoms, but unbeknownst to you, your body is functioning sub-optimally, and that afternoon tiredness or those red eyes, which you previously attributed to working too hard, may really be signs of mold toxicity.

If you don't pass the Visual Contrast Sensitivity test, you may then want to do a blood test for mycotoxins. One lab that does this type of testing is BioSign Laboratory Corporation: *BioSignLabs.com.*

After this, thoroughly and carefully inspect your home for mold and water leaks. Also, consider doing an ERMI test. If the ERMI reveals no harmful molds in your home, then you'll want to inspect your workplace for mold, and consider whether other places where you have worked or lived over the past several years have smelled musty or had water leaks.

Mold can remain in the body for years, so even if you haven't lived or worked in a moldy environment recently, your body may yet be harboring mold toxins from a home or work environment that you spent time in on a regular basis years ago.

Having mold in your home, in and of itself, doesn't mean that your body is being harmed by it. However, if ERMI or culture-plate testing reveals that mold is present, and you also suffer from undiagnosed symptoms and are not feeling well, it is worth doing further testing to find out whether mold toxins are the cause.

Symptoms of mold toxicity can be many and varied, and overlap with symptoms of other illnesses. Therefore, it's best to consult with a doctor who can distinguish mold illness from other types of disease. Common symptoms of mold illness include, but aren't limited to: fatigue, weakness, aches, muscle pain and cramps; headaches, light sensitivity, blurred vision, red eyes, sinus problems, cough, shortness of breath, abdominal pain, joint pain, memory and concentration problems, and mood swings.

In any case, it's never a good idea to live in a moldy home, so whether you feel good or not, consider removing all sources of mold from your living and/or work environment. This will help to ensure that you or your loved ones won't become sick in the future from it.

Detoxifying the Body of Mold and Mycotoxins

Removing mold and mycotoxins from the body can be a complicated endeavor. Therefore, as with heavy metal toxins, it's best to work with a naturopathic or integrative medical doctor who specializes in environmental or mold toxicity, if you suspect that you have mold illness. The details of mold detoxification therapy are beyond the scope of this book, so the information in this section should be treated only as a starting point for understanding how to remove mold toxins from the body.

We also recommend consulting the works of Ritchie Shoemaker, MD, which are found on the website: *Surviving Mold.com.* His books, *Surviving Mold: Life in an Era of Dangerous Buildings* and *Mold Warriors,* provide a more comprehensive understanding of mold toxicity and treatment.

Before you detoxify your body, you will first want to remove any mold from your home, workplace and anywhere else you spend a lot of time. It's not possible to fully recover from mold toxicity as long as you are being exposed to mold. Once you have remediated your environment, you can then begin the process of eliminating mold and its toxins from your body.

Fortunately, mold, like other types of toxins, can be effectively removed from the body, and the body restored to health if you have the right tools and are working with a qualified, competent, holistic physician.

It's important to note that separate treatments may be needed for mold and its mycotoxins. Mold is a live organism (a fungus) and should be eliminated first using antimicrobial remedies, and its toxins removed with powerful toxin binders. Banderol and Cumanda, which are herbal products made by NutraMedix (*NutraMedix.com*) are effective at killing fungi, as are Pau d'Arco extract and many other herbs, including tea-tree, clove, cinnamon, peppermint and rosemary. These are among the strongest natural antifungal remedies available on the market today.

Also, mold and other fungi cannot be successfully removed from the body as long as you are consuming foods that contain sugar or starch. This includes all grains, legumes, starchy veggies (such as potatoes), fruits, fruit juices, alcoholic beverages and vinegar, as well as most dairy products. Such foods encourage fungal growth and should be eliminated from your diet for eight to ten weeks, which is the amount of time that's usually required to effectively treat most fungal infections.

If you have severe mold toxicity or other health problems, however, you may need to maintain this diet and take antifungal remedies for a longer period of time. Dr. Cowden has developed an anti-fungal diet for his patients that can be found at:

ACIMConnect.com

When removing mycotoxins, not just any toxin binder will do. One of the most powerful and effective mycotoxin binders is the cholesterol-lowering drug, cholestyramine. This drug binds to bile in the gallbladder and prevents any fat-soluble toxins contained in the gallbladder from re-circulating throughout the body. Because cholestyramine is a drug, it can cause side effects, especially if you already have low cholesterol levels, and may be a better option only if you are seriously ill from mold toxins.

Also, according to America's Pharmacist™, Suzy Cohen, cholestyramine can suppress the body's absorption of fat-soluble vitamins. She says, "If you are using bile acid sequestrant drugs such as cholestyramine, you should supplement with key nutrients such as vitamin A, D, E and K. I recommend taking those daily, but at least four hours away from the drug. Failing to do so can lead to nutrient deficiencies that increase your risk for vision problems, suppressed immunity, osteoporosis and cardiovascular complications. Always weigh the risk-to-benefit (ratio) of medications, and if you need them, support your body by replenishing what the medication takes out." More on Suzy's work and the impact of drug-induced nutrient depletion can be found on her website: *DearPharmacist.com* and in her book, *Drug Muggers: Which Medications are Robbing Your Body of Essential Nutrients and How to Restore Them.*

For most people, better choices of toxin binders might be Galla chinensis powder, activated charcoal or CholestePure, a natural plant-based product. Richard Loyd, a PhD nutritionist in Seattle, recommends CholestePure to his clients. It's important to take these products at least two hours away from food and other supplements, since they also bind to these things.

Dr. Loyd has also found that ionic footbaths help his clients recover from mold toxicity. In his article, "Mold and Lyme Toxins," he describes how to make an inexpensive ionic footbath at home. This article can be found at: *RoyalRife.com/mold_toxins.pdf*

Banderol and Cumanda, which are herbal products made by NutraMedix (*Nutramedix.com*) are effective at killing fungi, as are Pau d'Arco extract and many other herbs, including tea-tree, clove, cinnamon, peppermint and rosemary.

Again, if you suspect that you have mold toxicity because you have found mold in your home or an ERMI test reveals high levels of mold toxins, and you also have some of the aforementioned symptoms, it's best to seek assistance from a naturopathic or integrative medical doctor experienced in treating environmental illness. These types of doctors can help you get those toxins out of your body, since mold toxin removal isn't really a do-it-yourself business!

Fortunately, mold, like other types of toxins, can be effectively removed from the body, and the body restored to health if you have the right tools and are working with a qualified, competent, holistic physician.

In Summary

By now you should have a pretty good idea about the broad range of environmental toxins to which we are all exposed daily, and how they affect—and infect—our bodies and homes. Hopefully, you understand that as part of the journey towards wellness, it's essential to remove as many of these toxins as possible and practice detoxification as a lifestyle if you want to be healthy and live long.

It's difficult for most people to enjoy vibrant health and well-being as long as their bodies are being plagued by a plethora of environmental toxins. These toxins are wreaking havoc upon even the strongest of people and are a major cause of most of the chronic and degenerative diseases that afflict our society.

Fortunately, the holistic medical community is continually coming up with new solutions for removing these toxins from our internal and external environments. Some of the most innovative and effective of these solutions have been presented in this book. We believe that by implementing at least some of them, you will enjoy better, more vibrant health, which in turn will equip you to enjoy life more fully and abundantly.

Further Reading and References

Food Toxins

Annual Report of the Pesticide Residues Committee. (2008) *Pesticide Residues Committee*. Retrieved on Sept. 2, 2013 from: *Pesticides.gov. uk/Resources/CRD/Migrated-Resources/Documents/P/PRC_Annual_Report 2008.pdf*

David, D., et al. (2004) Changes in USDA Food Composition Data for 43 Garden Crops, 1950 to 199. *Journal of the American College of Nutrition.* Vol. 23, No. 6 669-652

Fallon, S. The Right Price. *The Weston A. Price Foundation.* Retrieved on Sept. 22, 2013 from: *WestonAPrice.org/basics.*

Food Commission, UK. (Jan.-March, 2006) United Kingdom: Meat and dairy: Where have all the minerals gone? *Food Magazine.* Retrieved on December 1, 2011 from: *FoodComm.org.uk.*

Open Letter from World Scientists to All Governments Concerning GMOs. (2000) *Institute of Science and Society.* Retrieved on Sept. 12, 2013 from: *I-sis.org.uk/list.php.*

Pollan, M. (2009) *Food Rules.* New York, NY: Penguin Group.

Pollan, M. (2006) *The Omnivore's Dilemma.* New York, NY: Penguin Group.

Vogt R, Bennett D, Cassady D, Frost J, Ritz B, Hertz-Picciotto I. (2012, Nov. 9) Cancer and non-cancer health effects from food contaminant exposures for children and adults in California: a risk assessment. *Environ Health*; 11:83. doi: 10.1186/1476-069X-11-83.

United States: Vegetables Without Vitamins (2001, March) *Life Extension Magazine.* Retrieved on March 1, 2012 from: *LEF.org/ magazine/mag2001/mar2001_report_vegetables.html*

Toxins in Water

Pharmaceuticals in Drinking Water. *Philadelphia Water Department.* Retrieved on Sept. 2, 2013 from: *Phila.gov/water/Pharmaceuticals_ in_D.html*

Probe: Pharmaceuticals in Drinking Water. (2009, Feb. 11) *CBS News CBSNews.com/2100-204_162-3920454.html*

Toxins in Personal Care Products

Gordon, A. (2012, April 16) Toxic Personal Care Products Used Every Day. *Green Med Info.* Retrieved on Sept. 2, 2013 from: *GreenMedInfo. com/blog/toxic-personal-care-products-used-everyday*

Ji, S. (2013, May 7) Let Food Be Your Cosmetic: Coconut Oil Outperforms Dangerous Petroleum Body Care Products. *Green Med Info.* Retrieved on Sept. 2, 2013 from: *GreenMedInfo.com/blog/let-food-be-your- cosmetic-coconut-oil-outperforms-dangerous-petroleum-body-care*

Winter, R. (2009, Oct.) *A Consumer's Dictionary of Cosmetic Ingredients, 7th Edition*: Harmony Books.

Toxic Effects of Pharmaceutical Drugs

Estrogen plus progestin therapy and breast cancer in recently postmeno- pausal women. (2008, May 15) *Am J Epidemiol.*, 167(10):1207-16. doi: 10.1093/aje/kwn044. Epub 2008 Mar 27

Folkers K, Langsjoen P, Willis R, Richardson P, Xia LJ, Ye CQ, Tamagawa H. (1990, Nov). Lovastatin decreases coenzyme Q levels in humans. *Proc Natl Acad Sci* USA, 87(22):8931-4

Gullestad L, Oie E, Ueland T, Yndestad A, Aukrust P. (2007, Nov.) The role of statins in heart failure. *Fundam Clin Pharmacol.*, 21 Suppl 2:35-40.

Potgieter M, Pretorius E, Pepper MS. (2013, Mar) Primary and secondary coenzyme Q10 deficiency: the role of therapeutic supplementation. *Nutr Rev.*, 71(3):180-8. doi: 10.1111/nure.12011. Epub 2013 Jan 30.

Whitaker, J. It's Life, Not Depression. *Whitaker Wellness Medical Institute Medical Clinic.* Retrieved on Sept. 2, 2013 from: *WhitakerWellness. com/health-concerns/natural-treatments-for-depression/treatment- for-depression*

Heavy Metal Toxicity

Capo MA, Alonso CE, Sevil MB, Frejo MT. (1994) "In vitro" effects of methyl-mercury on the nervous system: a neurotoxicologic study. *J Environ Pathol Toxicol Oncol.*, 13(2):117-23.

Cutler, A. (1999, June) *Amalgam Illness: Diagnosis and Treatment.* Andrew Hall Cutler; 1st edition.

Gordon, G. and Brown, D. (2007) *Detox with Oral Chelation: Protecting Yourself from Lead, Mercury, & Other Environmental Toxins.* Petaluma, CA: Smart Publications.

Mania M, Wojciechowska-Mazurek M, Starska K, Rebeniak M, Postupolski J. (2012) Fish and seafood as a source of human exposure to methylmercury. *Rocz Panstw Zakl Hig.*, 63(3):257-64.

Shaw CA, Tomljenovic L. (2013 Jul) Aluminum in the central nervous system (CNS): toxicity in humans and animals, vaccine adjuvants, and autoimmunity. *Immunol Res.*,56(2-3):304-16. doi: 10.1007/s12026-013-8403-1.

Walton, JR. (2013, Jan. 1) Aluminum involvement in the progression of Alzheimer's disease. *J Alzheimer's Dis.*, 35(1):7-43. doi: 10.3233/JAD-121909.

Radiation

Mangano, Joseph J., Janette D. Sherman (2013, March) Elevated airborne beta levels in Pacific/West Coast US States and trends in hypothyroidism among newborns after the Fukushima nuclear meltdown. *OJPed*, Vol.3 No. 1DOI. 10.4236/ojped.2013.31001

Mangano, Joseph J., Janette D Sherman. (2012) An unexpected mortality increase in the United States follows arrival of the radioactive plume from Fukushima: is there a correlation? *Int J Health Serv.*;42(1):47-64

Dental Foci Infections/Root Canals

Hal Huggins' DDS website: *HugginsAppliedHealing.com*

Huggins, H. (2010) Root Canal Dangers. *The Weston A. Price Foundation.* Retrieved on March 18, 2012 from: *WestonAPrice.org/dentistry/root-canal-dangers*

Huggins (1999) *Uninformed Consent: The Hidden Dangers in Dental Care.* Newburyport, MA: Hampton Roads Publications.

New DNA Study Confirms Decades-Old Research that Root Canals Contain Toxic Bacterium that may be the 'Root' Cause of Many Diseases. *Toxic Element Research Foundation.* Retrieved on Sept. 2, 2013 from: *TERFInfo.com/Files/Root%20Canal%20News%20Release_2.pdf*

DETOXIFICATION PRODUCTS

Biomat: *BioMat.com*

Chi Machine: *ChiMachine4u.com*

Heel homeopathic detoxification remedies: *Heel.com*

NutraMedix: *NutraMedix.com*

Pekana homeopathic detoxification remedies: *Pekana.com*

HOUSEHOLD TOXINS

Air Purification Products

Austin Air hepa filters: *AustinAir.com*

Nikken air filters: *Nikken.com/product/technology/air-wellness*

Carpet

Anderson, J. (1997) Reactions to Carpet Emissions. A Case Series. *Journal of Nutritional and Environmental Medicine* ; 7: 177-185.

DDT. Pesticide Action Network. Retrieved on Sept. 2, 2013 from: *PANNA.org/resources/specific-pesticides/DDT*

Michael, D. Toxic Carpet: Dangerous Toxins that Live in Your Carpeting. Retrieved on Sept. 2, 2013 from: *GreenAndHealthy.info/toxiccarpeting.html*

Electromagnetic Radiation

Biological effects from electromagnetic field exposure and public exposure standards (2008 Feb). *Biomed Pharmacother.* ;62(2):104-9. doi: 10.1016/j.biopha.2007.12.004. Epub 2007 Dec 31. Retrieved on Sept. 2, 2013 from: *NCBI.nlm.nih.gov/pubmed/18242044*

Carlo, G. (2007). The Hidden Dangers of Cell Phone Radiation. *Life Extension Magazine.* Retrieved on March 7, 2012 from: *LEF.org/magazine/mag2007/aug2007_report_cellphone_radiation_01.htm*

Cherry, Neil. (2002-2005). Epidemiological Studies of Enhanced Brain/CNS Cancer Incidence and Mortality from EMR and EMF Exposures. *Lincoln University,* Canterbury, NZ. Retrieved on Sept. 2, 2013 from: *NeilCherry.com/documents/90_s1_EMR_Brain_cancer_paper09-02.pdf*

Cherry, Neil. (2002-2005). Evidence that EMF/EMR Causes Leukaemia/Lymphoma in Adults and Children. *Lincoln University*, Canterbury, NZ. Retrieved on Sept. 2, 2013 from: *ResearchArchive. lincoln.ac.nz/bitstream/10182/4005/1/90_s5_EMR_Leukaemia_ Review_Paper.pdf*

Crofton, K. (2010) *Wireless Radiation Rescue.* Global Wellbeing Books

Del Sol, J. (Producer and Director). (2013, Sept. 5) *Take Back Your Power.* Available from: *TakeBackYourPower.net/*

Draper, G. (2005, June 2) Childhood cancer in relation to distance from high voltage power lines in England and Wales: a case-control study. *BMJ; 330 doi: DX.doi.org/10.1136/bmj.330.7503.1290.* Retrieved on Sept. 2, 2013 from: *BMJ.com/content/330/7503/1290.*

Electromagnetic Health (website of Camilla Rees, MBA): *ElectroMagneticHealth.org*

EMR Stop. (2010).Transcript Interview with Dr. Thomas M. Rau of the Paracelsus Clinic. Retrieved on Jan. 12, 2011 from: *ERMStop.org/ index.php?option=com_content&view=article&id=139:transcript-interview-with-dr-thomas-m-rau-of-the-swiss-paracelsus-clinic&catid= 6:K.* (2010) *ERMStop.org*

Fauteux, A. Electromagnetic Intolerance Elucidated. *EMFacts Consultancy.* Retrieved on Feb. 7, 2011 from: *EMFacts.com/2012/01/electro-magnetic-intolerance-elucidated/*

French Association for Research in Therapeutics against Cancer: *ARTAC.info*

Havas, M. (Producer) (2011, Dec. 4) *Wi-Fi in Schools is Safe: True or False?* Retrieved on Sept. 2, 2013 from: *YouTube.com/ watch?v=6v75sKAUFdc*

Ober, C., Sinatra, S. and Zucker, M. (2010) *Earthing: The Most Important Health Discovery Ever?* Laguna Beach, CA: Basic Health Publications.

Rees, Camilla. (2009) *Public Health SOS; The Shadow Side of The Wireless Revolution.* Charlestown, SC: Create Space.

The Institute of Building Biology + Ecology Neubeuern: *BauBiologie.de/ site/english.php*

Pets

Koo, I. (2009, Feb.) Toxoplasmosis Congenital Disease. *About.com.* Retrieved on Sept. 15, 2013 from: *InfectiousDiseases.about.com/od/ diseasesbyname/a/Toxoplasmosis.htm*

EMR REMEDIATION PRODUCTS

Earthing products: *EarthingInstitute.net*

EMR Protection Products: *LessEMF.com/gauss.html*

EMF Safety Store: *EMFSafetyStore.com*

Graham-Stetzer filters: *StetzerElectric.com*

Memon products: *MemonYourHarmony.com*

Smart Meters

Stan Hartman, RadSafe, Boulder, Colorado: *RadSafe.net*

Stop Smart Meters! *StopSmartMeters.org*

Mold Toxins and Mold Illness

Mold, a health alert. (1999, Dec. 5) *USA Weekend.* Retrieved on Sept. 2, 2013 from: *159.54.226.237/99_issues/991205/991205mold.html*

Schaller, J. (2006) *Mold Illness and Mold Remediation Made Simple (Discount Black & White Edition): Removing Mold Toxins from Bodies and Sick Buildings.* Tampa, FL: Hope Academic Press.

Schaller, James, MD: *PersonalConsult.com*

Shoemaker, R. (2011) *Surviving Mold: Life in the Era of Dangerous Buildings.* Otter Bay Books

Shoemaker, R., et al. (2010) *Policy Holders of America: Research Committee Report on Diagnosis and Treatment of Chronic Inflammatory Response Syndrome Caused by Exposure to the Interior Environment of Water-Damaged Buildings:* Pokomoke, Maryland. Retrieved on May 1, 2012 from: *SurvivingMold.com/legal-resources/publications/ poa-position-statement-paper.*

Shoemaker, R. (2005) *Mold Warriors.* Baltimore, MD: Gateway Press, Inc.

Shoemaker, Ritchie, MD: *SurvivingMold.com*

Solfrizzo M, et al. (2001) In vitro and in vivo studies to assess the effectiveness of cholestyramine as a binding agent for fumonisins. *Mycopathologia,* 147-153. Retrieved on April 10, 2012 from: *USMold Physician.com/articles/comparingmoldtoxinbinders.html.*

Resources For Mold Testing

Environmental Health Center of Dallas: *EHCD.com*

ERMI-DNA Mold Testing: *ERMIMoldTest.com*

Real Time Labs: *RealTimeLab.com*

Mold Toxin Removal Products

Cholestepure: *PureEncapsulations.com/itemdy00.asp?T1=CHP1*

NutraMedix' Banderol and other products: *NutraMedix.com*

Thieves' oil: *SecretOfThieves.com*

About the Authors

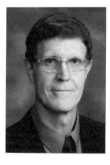

William Lee Cowden, MD, MD(H), is a U.S. board-certified cardiologist and internist internationally renowned and recognized for his knowledge and skill in practicing and teaching integrative medicine.

He is chairman of the scientific advisory board and academy professor for the Academy of Comprehensive Integrative Medicine (ACIM). ACIM is dedicated to shifting the healthcare paradigm toward wellness by training and supporting practitioners in a variety of holistic health disciplines, conducting research, and implementing therapeutic innovations to create a new global wellness care community.

Dr. Cowden has pioneered successful treatments for a myriad of diseases, including chronic fatigue syndrome, cancer, autism, fibromyalgia, heart disease, Lyme disease, and others.

In addition to treating thousands of patients, Dr. Cowden travels and teaches integrative medicine nationally and internationally in countries such as Mexico, Brazil, Peru, Guatemala, Germany, the Czech Republic, Japan, China, Taiwan, England, the Netherlands, Austria, Australia, Norway, Curaçao, the Dominican Republic, Singapore and Malaysia. He is also a member of the Lyme and Autism Foundation scientific advisory board.

Dr. Cowden is the author or co-author of many publications, including the following books: *Insights into Lyme Disease Treatment* (2009); *Longevity, An Alternative Medicine Definitive Guide* (2001); *Cancer Diagnosis: What to do Next* (2000); and the best-selling *An Alternative Medicine Definitive Guide to Cancer* (1997).

Although Dr. Cowden was initially trained in traditional, allopathic medicine, early on in his career he realized that this type of medicine often not only didn't get his patients well, but frequently failed to bring them to a place of wholeness so that their illnesses wouldn't recur. So he quickly expanded his knowledge, experience and medical practice to include natural, non-toxic, holistic solutions for wellness.

More than a holistic physician, however, Dr. Cowden is also a sensitive educator who teaches his patients lifestyle, emotional and spiritual strategies for living well so that they can go beyond wellness to wholeness—in body, mind and spirit.

More information about Dr. Cowden and his work can be found on the Academy of Comprehensive Integrative Medicine website: *ACIMConnect.com.*

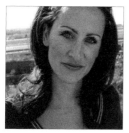 **Connie Strasheim** is a medical researcher and writer who has experienced the hardships of chronic illness firsthand through her near decade-long battle with Lyme disease and chronic fatigue syndrome. Besides co-authoring the books in this series, she is the author of five books on holistic treatments for disease, including the best-selling *Insights Into Lyme Disease Treatment: Thirteen Lyme-Literate Health Care Practitioners Share Their Healing Strategies (2009); Beyond Lyme Disease: Healing The Underlying Causes of Chronic Illness in People with Borreliosis and Co-Infections* (2012); *Defeat Cancer: 15 Doctors of Integrative and Naturopathic Medicine Tell You How* (2010); *Healing Chronic Illness: By His Spirit, Through His Resources* (2010); and *The Lyme Disease Survival Guide: Physical, Lifestyle and Emotional Strategies for Healing (2008).*

Through her battle with severe chronic illness, Connie has learned that attaining wellness isn't just about eliminating infections, detoxifying the body or balancing the hormones—it's about addressing all the factors that caused the body to break down in the first place. These include all environmental, psycho-emotional, lifestyle and spiritual issues that cause or contribute to damage, discontent and—ultimately—"dis-ease" in the body, mind and spirit.

She has also learned, through her experience and research, that in order to be well—never mind whole—in today's world fraught with stress and toxicity, many tools are required. In this book series, *The Journey to Wellness,* she and Dr. Cowden share some of these tools.

More information about Connie's work can be found at: *ConnieStrasheim.com.*

How to Contact *William Lee Cowden, MD, MD(H)* and *Connie Strasheim*

Dr. Cowden is retired from private practice and no longer sees patients of his own. He now embraces his passion to bring to health professionals across the world his successful, natural and non-invasive techniques for reversing advanced cancer, autism, Lyme disease, atherosclerosis and many other chronic diseases. These are techniques that he has pioneered over his many years of practice. Dr. Cowden has previously co-authored two books on alternative treatments for cancer as well as a book on Longevity and has contributed to several other books. He is currently the Chairman of the Scientific Advisory Board for the Academy of Comprehensive Integrative Medicine. As part of his role at the Academy, he produces online courses and does teaching webinars on integrative medicine.

He is available to speak at conferences and for interviews, and to teach health practitioners at their clinical practices. To discuss speaking, teaching or interview opportunities with Dr. Cowden, please contact the Academy of Comprehensive Integrative Medicine at: *info@ACIMConnect.com*.

Connie Strasheim is the author of seven books on holistic wellness, including Lyme disease, cancer, and spiritual healing. She is available for teaching and speaking engagements as well as media interviews. You can invite Connie to your webinar, conference, radio or TV show by contacting her at: *Connie9824@aol.com*.

She shares her life experiences with people who have chronic health conditions through her blog: *ConnieStrasheim.blogspot.com*. In addition, she hosts a public bi-monthly prayer conference call group, the details of which can be found on her FB page: *FaceBook.com/ Connie.Strasheim*. For more information on Connie and her work, visit: *ConnieStrasheim.com*.